TANTRIC SEX

A Complete Guide for Couples to the Ancient Tantric Art of Sex. Kamasutra, Tantric Massage, Benefits and Tips to Get in Touch with the Tantric Zone and Revitalize Your Sex Life

Paisley Macy

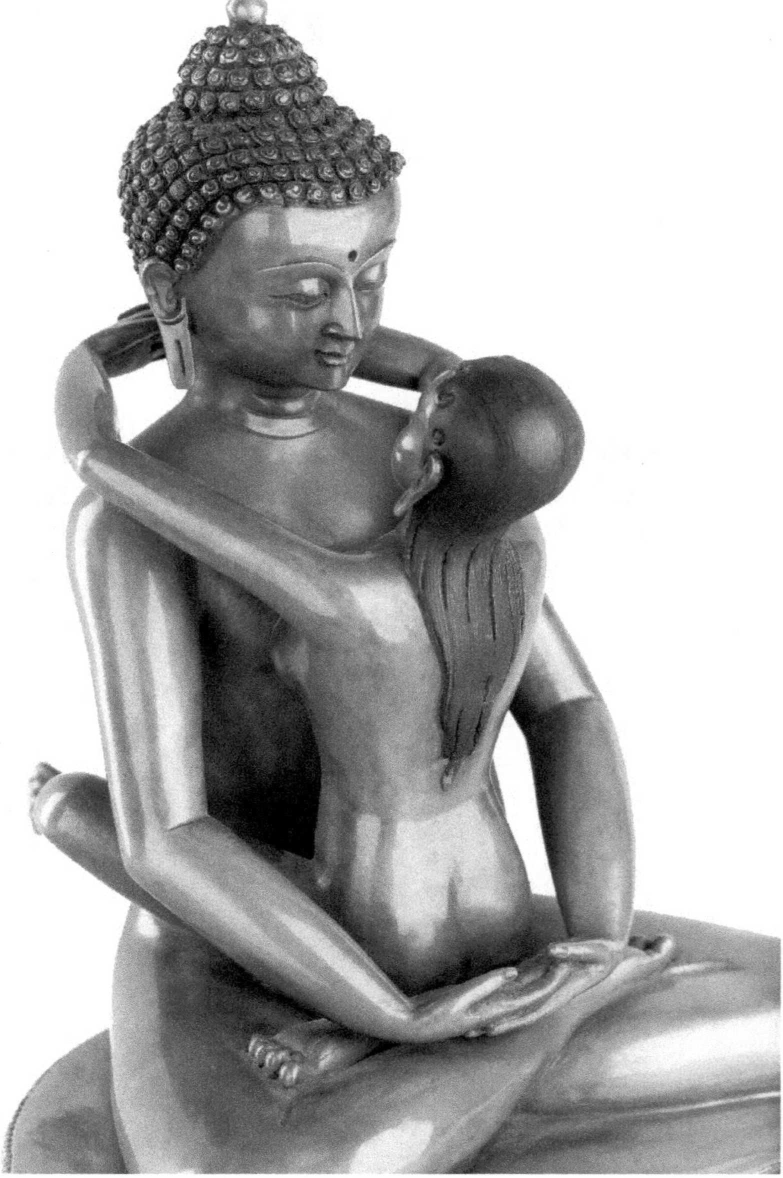

The following Book is reproduced below with the goal of providing information that is as accurate and reliable as possible. Regardless, purchasing this Book can be seen as consent to the fact that both the publisher and the author of this book are in no way experts on the topics discussed within and that any recommendations or suggestions that are made herein are for entertainment purposes only. Professionals should be consulted as needed prior to undertaking any of the action endorsed herein.

This declaration is deemed fair and valid by both the American Bar Association and the Committee of Publishers Association and is legally binding throughout the United States.

The information in the following pages is broadly considered a truthful and accurate account of facts and as such, any inattention, use, or misuse of the information in question by the reader will render any resulting actions solely under their purview. There are no scenarios in which the publisher or the original author of this work can be in any fashion deemed liable for any hardship or damages that may befall them after undertaking information described herein.

Additionally, the information in the following pages is intended only for informational purposes and should thus be thought of as universal. As befitting its nature, it is presented without assurance regarding its prolonged validity or interim quality. Trademarks that are mentioned are done without written consent and can in no way be considered an endorsement from the trademark holder.

[illegible] constitute the [illegible] [illegible] of the [illegible] [illegible] which the publisher [illegible] [illegible] that may [illegible] the [illegible] described [illegible].

Additionally, the [illegible] in the following pages is [illegible] for [illegible] informational purposes and should [illegible] be thought [illegible]. As [illegible] it is presented without [illegible] regarding [illegible] validity [illegible] [illegible] that are mentioned [illegible] done without [illegible] consent and can [illegible] be considered [illegible] endorsement from the [illegible].

Table of Contents

Introduction

There are clouded notions when it comes to the history of Tantra. However, the associations that experts have come up with, which seem the most likely, are that Tantra is related to spirituality that early Hindus practiced over 6000 years ago.

There has also been speculation about whether early Buddhists practiced Tantra.

Given that these are philosophies and religions, one may wonder what the connection is between them and sexual activity.

However, the answer lies in what we know to be energy. Every human being has energy, as has every living thing.

Tantra is the joining of energies in the most delightful way possible so that sex and massage are not just indulgent pleasures but are the joining of two energies to feel a higher sense of fulfillment.

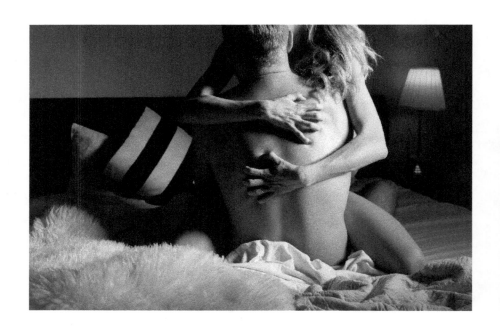

Chapter 1.
Basic Principle of Tantric Sex

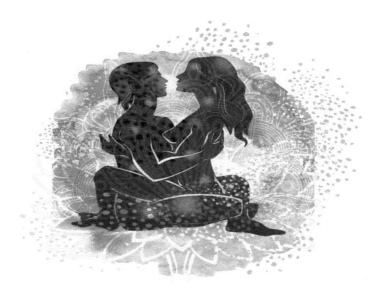

Different Steps for Lovemaking

In the foreplay, as well as during the sexual act, one uses a variety of actions. According to tantric sex, the various actions involved would consist of the following:

• Bites – When done correctly, biting can be pleasurable! This isn't the painful kind of biting; make sure your partner is well-aroused and start with little nibbles around erogenous and sensitive zones before working your way up to hard bites that can leave marks.

• Scratches – The tips of your fingers and blunt nails can be quite sensuous. Ladies, be careful of long nails, so you don't cause too much pain! Again, go slowly and make sure you're well aroused to add to the experience instead of being painful.

• Kissing – This requires no explanation, but kissing is a must for any sexual activity! The lips contain a huge number of nerve endings, which is why they're so sensitive. So make sure to pepper your partner's body with kisses!

• Embraces – Rubbing skin against skin is one of the most erotic things you will ever feel. Sex isn't just about rubbing your genitals together; it's a way of experiencing a human connection, even if it's just a one-night stand. An embrace between partners will heighten the emotional and physical experience, so don't be afraid to have naked cuddle time!

• Rubbing – Just dragging your fingers over your partner's erogenous zones and softly rubbing against them is more arousing than you can imagine. Use your fingers, the flat of your palms, the tips of your toes, and even your tongue!

• Grips – Gripping your partner tight is usually quite arousing, but make sure it's safe and consensual! Rough sex gets a lot of people going, after all.

• Different sex positions – Trying out different sexual positions will help you explore your dynamic as a couple. Who likes being on top, who enjoys giving up control, etc., and all those ideas that define you as a couple can take place only if you experiment!

• Combination of poses – Try out different poses and work your style of sex that is individualistic to you! There's no right way to have sex; just find what works for you and your partner!

Actions Involving the Side of the Woman

Actions Involving the Male Penis

• Locating and caressing sexually sensitive areas of the body – Find the erogenous zones; the misconception is that it's only the genital and sexual organs that bring pleasure. That's not true; each person has different spots on their sensitive body, and rubbing/kissing/licking/sucking these areas will help.

• Sucking – The action of sucking on the skin can be quite arousing if you do it right. It provides friction and arouses; start small with licking around the sensitive skin, slowly press your whole mouth and suck gently.

• Slapping – An aspect of rough sex, you have to be certain your partner enjoys it! Some people are put off by too much roughness in their sex lives, so be careful. Spanking, for instance, is something that a lot of people enjoy; the adrenalin rush brings with it endorphins that give you a high like nothing else! But be careful – make sure you both want it before you jump into it.

• Hair movements – Using your hair is a very arousing thing. It's ticklish, it's feather-like, and it can arouse; men's stubble and beard can be very exciting when rubbed against sensitive areas. And a woman's long hair can feel very sensuous.

Exciting The Nerves

• Using the tongue – In sex, your tongue is your greatest weapon, along with your fingers. Its soft, yet rough texture arouses better than anything else, so lick and play with the tongue as much as you can!

Eroticism of The Embrace

The Kama Sutra categorizes embraces as one of the eight types. It is a part of the foreplay. Depending on the approach and intention, we have different classes of embraces.

a. First, we will examine two kinds of embraces between people who do not often talk to each other. In the touching embrace, the man will approach the woman citing some reason or the other and then touch her body with his own.

b. If the woman turns or bends towards a man as if to complete some other action and "pierces" the man with her breasts, and the man in return takes them with his own hands, it becomes a piercing embrace. This they can do with ease in some lonely place.

c. Once the lovers have become familiar with one another and move and talk freely, then there is the possibility of the rubbing embrace. While walking side by side, the lovers rub their bodies against each other. This is the rubbing embrace.

d. The pressing embrace has similarities to this. In the pressing embrace, one of the lovers will press against the other's body and then lean their bodies into a wall or a pillar. These two types of embraces' intentions are apparent to the lovers since they are lovers for a long time.

e. Next, depending on the type of hold and stance, we have another four embraces. This classification is into two physical and two mental analogies. First, two are the twining creeper and the tree climber. The second two refer to food and tastes. One refers to combining sesame seeds with rice, while the second refers to the joining of milk and water.

f. The first two embraces described here take place when the man is standing. In practice, the woman pulls the head of the man down to hers and entwines her body around his, and with a longing look in her eyes, she looks up eagerly for the kiss. Her mouth begins to suck in air, and an audible sound escapes from her lips.

This is the twining creeper. If she grips his shoulder with an arm while gripping his back with the other arm and places her foot over his, she is doing the climbing the tree embrace. Her mouth longs for his kiss, and she places her other leg over his thigh.

g. The next embrace takes place between lovers who like each other so much that they do not think of love or hurt. This embrace will occur when she is sitting on his lap or in front of him. They seem to enter each other's body and pass into one being.

h. The last embrace occurs when they are sleeping on the bed. They hold each other so tightly that their arms seem to rub against the other all the while.

Premature Ejaculation

In some of the sex fantasies of men, we see that they desire a beautiful woman to approach him and give him a blowjob. Just like that, she unzips his trousers and gives him oral sex. She sucks on his penis until he ejaculates and then walks away.

This places enormous stress on women who like to proceed slowly or do not like to take it in the mouth. It also makes men ejaculate prematurely.

Another reason for premature ejaculation is the lack of exercise. A regular 9-5 job with set routines makes the man a machine. He does things without any real thinking.

When he climbs into bed, his mind is still stagnant. His movements lack coordination with his emotions. His emotions once copulation begins run haywire, and soon, he has premature ejaculation.

The reason is that he feels too much excitement too quickly; there is not enough time for a slow, steady buildup of sexual energy. One more reason for this failure on the part of men during intercourse is due to improper nutrition.

When you take food containing fried stuff like fried chicken or meat and sugary things like carbonated water and pastries, the metabolism becomes hyperactive. It recognizes only these glucose-containing items and the saturated fat items as real food.

The rate of your metabolism gets set to this frequency. What happens is that the cholesterol content of the body increases.

The flow of blood becomes sluggish. The rate at which oxygen goes to different parts of the body slows down. The overall functioning of the body slows down.

When you ingest a lot of glucose too soon, the blood leaps on this energy source, and, being a simple sugar, consumes it at once. The energy level spikes. But then, being simple sugars, all of it soon disappears. The energy level plummets. This leads to craving, and you begin to eat more fried and sugary stuff. A little intake of high-calorie foods like jaggery, (Cane sugar), banana, and papaya, along with milk, will help hugely before (and after) sex. Overdoing it kills.

Added to this, people with medical conditions like urethritis, elevated blood pressure, underactive thyroids, and diabetes will suffer from the problem of premature ejaculation. Problems with erection are common when your metabolism is not in peak condition.

Any condition that slows down the flow of blood or semen will result in premature ejaculation or imperfect erection.

Use the chakra method to raise your consciousness to a higher plane of interaction. Be aware of the various reasons, however, and take the proper steps. For instance, if you are diabetic, be sure to take your diabetic medicines.

Meditation will help you become mentally strong. You can control your emotions and energy flow since you realize what it is and what it does.

Oral Sex

Cunnilingus is what you do with your mouth, lips, and tongue to excite your partner during lovemaking. This act, when the female undergoes oral excitation by her partner, is what we call cunnilingus. The male uses his tongue and lips to excite the G-spot (clitoris) of his sex partner.

Begin by using small sucking motions with the lips to open the vagina to the delicate sensations. At first, you will see that her vagina is not responsive. Use your nose and lips to pull at the parting.

Keep sucking and licking the edges. Use your arms to grip her buttocks. You can also choose to gently and slowly send one finger up and down her anus. This optional step may take a long time, and lubrication such as saliva or sexual lubrication products may be needed.

This may not work for all people. However, it begins to excite her once you get your finger deep in her anus. Do anything that pleases you both, go wherever your sexual fantasy takes you.

When her vagina begins to open to you, you will see her legs opening up and widening. Now use longer and deeper licks with your tongue. Get inside her vagina and suck up to her upper portion. This will begin to stimulate her clitoris. The clitoris is a flap of skin that is present on the top of the vagina. If you rub this, she will get super excited.

Once she begins to sigh and moan, then you can begin sucking vigorously. Send the tongue once in a while deep into her vagina to excite her further. Once the Shakti (feminine energy) begins to increase, then you have an easy ride. This first portion is difficult work.

This cunnilingus makes the woman open up as it stirs her nerves and makes her eager to participate in the copulation.

This alternative to full-body caressing is more intimate and direct, and it helps you establish a close connection with her. The copulation becomes more intense.

Like a man, the woman also comes prematurely sometimes if you do not give her a good vaginal licking. Lick it and suck on it until she ejaculates. Once this occurs, she becomes prepared for the next stage of sexual intercourse.

Fellatio

This is the oral sex equivalent that a woman gives to a man. This has particular significance in helping the man avoid premature ejaculation.

Once the man comes when the woman gives him a blowjob, it removes the top chakra (Muladhara). It opens and begins to rise to the top to meet Shiva (masculine energy), the final state of existence.

The man has no more urge to come and so reaches his full orgasm without any premature ejaculation. This is possible between a man and a man too. The method of giving a blowjob will consist of the following steps: First, take the limp penis in the mouth.

Then she sucks on it. She uses alternate licking of the tip of the penis with her tongue. This makes the man super excited. The more she licks the tip of the penis, the harder the penis becomes.

When she does this, the chakra passes from the pubic zone to the next higher zone, which is the void. Here, he caresses her hair and breasts to move out of her zone to the next chakra.

The energy level interacts, and the external world closes out. Since the man begins from the lower Muladhara (chakra), he ejaculates, releasing his pent-up energy without any transition. Now, his chakra moves up; he no longer has any need to ejaculate.

Depending on the girl's stimulation, his energy transition takes him to a higher level of interaction. Sucking on the penis, the woman begins to get the energy vibes from the man. He is eager to transcend to the higher plane from where he can descend on the woman.

She uses her fingers to gently scratch or pinches his scrotum or balls and thighs. This makes his senses deviate, and he begins to moan and sigh.

When she hears this, she renews her efforts to sucking his penis with renewed energy. She moves her head up and down the shaft and uses her tongue to caress it.

Now and then, she licks the end of the penis so that he gets a shiver of excitement running up his spine. His energy levels ascend. Then he comes and is ready for the next step of lovemaking. He is now removed from premature ejaculation worries.

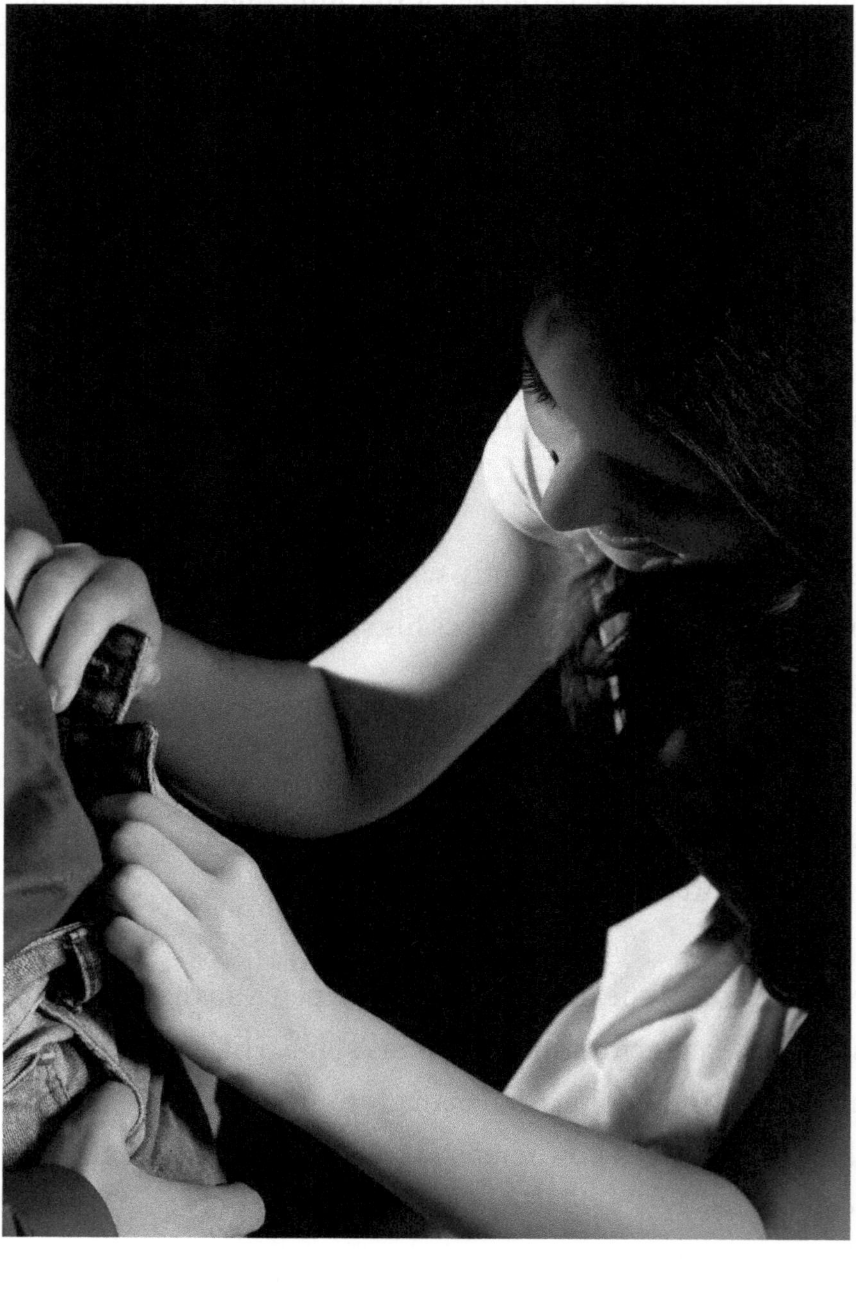

Chapter 2.

Difference between Kama Sutra and Tantric Sex

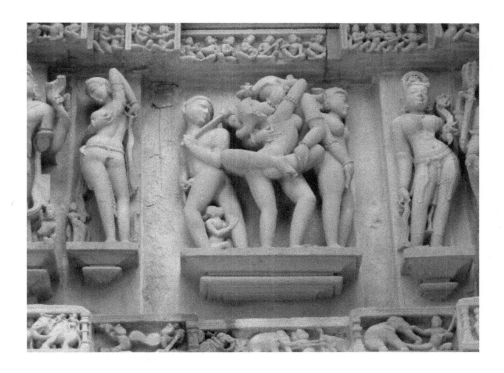

People often perceive that Kama Sutra and Tantric Sex are the same. It could be because both are part of an ancient sensual ritual that focuses on providing spiritual and sexual guidance to achieve a higher form of ecstasy.

They are, however, two different ideals. For one, Tantra is a mid-eastern Philosophy dealing with chakra points to enhance emotions and feelings. At the same time, Kama Sutra is an old eastern philosophy that focuses more on sexual positions. This chapter attempts to differentiate and compare these two ideas and how it will benefit our sex lives.

Knowing Kama Sutra

Kama Sutra is one of the earliest Hindu Love Manuals known. This is a list compiled by an Indian sage, Vatsyayana, depicting a compendium of love-customs and social norms in Northern India during his time.

His manual offers different scenarios of interactions couples are capable of having in lovemaking. He also offered several positions in which couples can enjoy during the activity.

Unlike Tantra, which was specifically written for a certain group of believers, Kama Sutra was written for the wealthy male city-dwellers. It was specifically written to provide sexual pleasure to the upper half of the society and never for the masses.

While Tantra explains the importance of sex with a partner as a part of transferring sexual energy to become a path to enlightenment, Kama Sutra mainly focuses on providing enjoyment, particularly to a man. Kama Sutra also mentions information about sex with more than one woman.

It was also thoroughly explained that Tantric Sex is a sacred ritual, a representation of the gods in copulation to reach enlightenment and create the cycle of death and rebirth.

While sex is valued as a sexual duty in Kama Sutra, on the other hand, it is still thoroughly expressed that the purpose of the transcript is entirely for pleasure and does not involve any meditation and reflection as compared to Tantric Sex.

Although it was thoroughly expressed that Tantric Sex and Kama Sutra are different ideologies, Tantra's main principles for positions are still dependent on the latter. The five main principles of Tantric lovemaking positions are based on Kama Sutra.

These are the following:

- Man on top

- Woman on top

- Seated positions

- Woman and man on their sides, face to face

- Woman with her back to the man

Comparing Side by Side

In the table below, you will see the major similarities and differences between Kama Sutra and Tantric Sex and how its difference matters to those who practice it.

Issue	Kama Sutra	Tantric Sex
Purpose	Provide sexual Pleasure to practitioners	To use sexual energy as a path to enlightenment
Who is it made for	Wealthy men in the City	Sadhaka Practitioners
The focus of the Manual	Different positions and strategies to provide sexual Pleasure	Integration of meditation and exercise to reach the highest form of ecstasy

Partner Involvement	May be applied to more than one woman	Focuses on one partner only
Positions	Involves plenty of positions aimed to provide enjoyment	Aims position to reach the highest form of orgasm; covers five Kama Sutra positions as the basic principle of Tantric Love Making positions

Difference Between Tantra and Kama Sutra

Many people are under the misconception that Tantra and Kama Sutra are the same things. This is not the case. Kama Sutra focuses on pleasure.

Tantra, on the other hand, focuses on the spiritual aspect. This misconception stems from the early days when some Tantras (Tantrikas) used the energy produced from sexualized group rituals to achieve enlightenment and magical powers (known as siddhis).

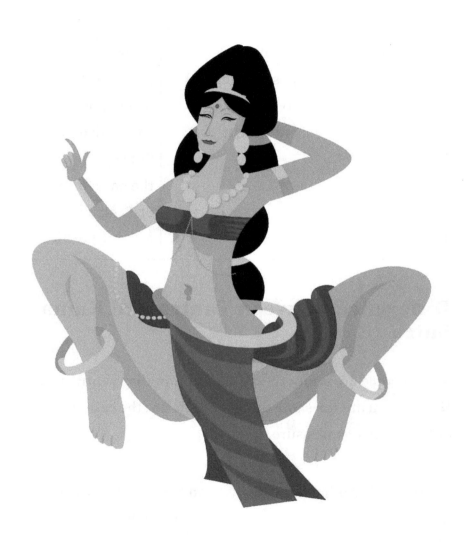

Tantra embraces sex as a sacred act, both inside and outside of marriage. It magnifies consciousness and releases it beyond that of our suppressive conditioning.

Tantric ideology regards sexual energy as an assistant to reach full spiritual enlightenment. The word Tantra means to weave. Tantra is more dedicated to the seven chakras and both the physical and mental aspects of each.

Kama Sutra is an ancient Indian Sanskrit exposition that discusses the nature of love, family life, and other aspects of human life's pleasure-oriented functions.

The word sutra means to teach. An example of this is modern Yoga. There is a teacher who tells people which positions to do. The original Kama Sutra book was written between the second and fourth centuries ACE by Vatsyayana.

In the book, he explained how to obtain a wife, her duties and privileges, the relations with other men's wives, and several other aspects of daily life. Approximately 20 percent is about sexual positions.

Mainly, it discusses what triggers desire, how to sustain it, and how and when it is good or bad. According to Kama Sutra, there are four goals to life: virtuous living, prosperity through materialistic possessions, desire, and liberation.

The terminology he used in the book is context-specific. Sexual intercourse is called Yoga, while to him, Tantra was meant as a method or technique.

The word Yantra meant a dildo or some other artificial device used for lovemaking. There are no Tantrikas that are similar to Kama Sutra.

One common Kama Sutra position is the 69 position, which is oral mutual honoring. When couples engage in this simultaneously, it can ignite internal energy that explodes throughout the body.

It creates an animalistic appetite that is extremely powerful. There are three variations to the 69 position.

Flowering Fern

The woman gets on top of the male, lowers her Yoni to his lips, and then bends down to welcome his lingam (penis) with her mouth. The female has two options: she can kneel with her knees on either side of his head or slide down, pressing her entire body against his.

Chapter 3.
Introduction to Tantric Sex

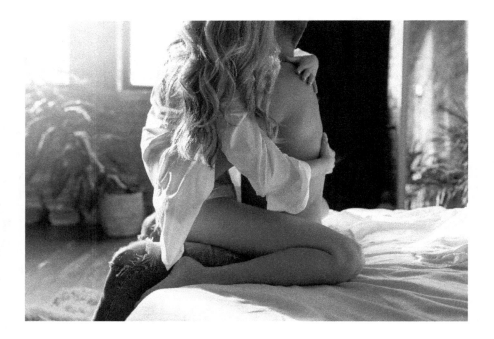

Many introduced Tantra to the Western world. Like Crowley, some failed to highlight the vital and spiritual aspects of the tradition, while others were more successful in bringing about widespread knowledge about the nature of Tantra.

But since Tantra was openly presented to the masses, many people have taken it upon themselves to introduce the tradition the right way.

And that is what we would like to accomplish here: to correctly introduce you to Tantra with the knowledge we have gained.

Who Doesn't Like Sex?

Most people, if not all, are excited about the idea – or interested in – sex. However, there is often limited openness when it comes to talking about sex.

Usually, people converse in hushed tones, afraid that someone might pick up on their conversation and immediately (and falsely, might we add) come to the conclusion that they have eavesdropped on a conversation between a bunch of perverts.

It truly is mind-boggling when you think that sex is enjoyed in so many ways – and even depicted in many ways through the visual medium. And yes, we are once again talking about porn. According to certain data, porn accounts for nearly 30% of all Internet traffic (Fight the New Drug, 2019).

We are exposed to sex and sexual references in so many ways. From movies to TV shows to even video games, sex has become an oft-referenced part of our lives. Yet the conversation surrounding it feels like people talk about a secret plan to destroy the whole world.

Tantra, on the other hand, refuses to keep the conversations surrounding sex a clandestine activity. Because of this open approach to discussing sex, it is because it tackles various aspects of the topic wisely.

Sexuality is viewed as a sacred activity in Tantra that expresses more than just physical pleasures. Sex becomes an intimate gesture and another form of human communication. Lovers using Tantric principles honor and respect each other, as though they were divine beings.

Each individual engaged in a sexual act is treated as an equal. No one is superior. Lovemaking becomes an act so profound that it aims to create a unity between lovers and a blissful state of consciousness.

Through such belief systems, Tantra considers sex as energy and the male and female forms as two parts of a greater whole.

Mars and Venus

You might have heard of people, life coaches, relationship advice books, and self-help gurus talk about men from Mars while women are from Venus. It is a symbolic way of telling people that men and women are completely different. Popular ideas often try to place men and women on opposite sides to understand them individually.

But Tantra finds a better solution when it comes to men and women. Rather than think of them as two sides of the same coin, it considers them a pair, like a yin and a yang symbol.

This idea creates a sense of harmony and encourages people to truly understand their partners. Rather than thinking that their partners are different, which only serves to build walls between people and reinforce the idea that the opposite gender is difficult to understand, Tantra's idea of pairs aims not just to create a bridge between men and women to strengthen that bridge.

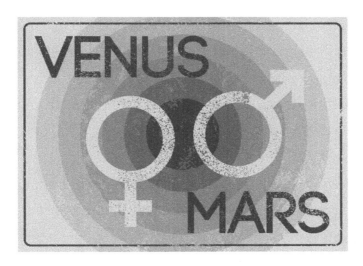

When you think about it, the idea of pairs is present in nature and surrounds us all. Day and night, light and darkness, the Earth and the sky, and water and fire are not contradictory elements, but forces complement each other.

Water is a force to douse the fire, a cure for the rage that fire creates. However, think about it this way. Water created life on Earth, which eventually evolved into early human beings, who then discovered fire to sustain life. Fire allowed humans to migrate to any part of the world.

No more did they have to suffer the relentless attacks of predators. They could survive in regions with colder climates. The fire also allowed humans to cook food, which is vital for their very survival.

Eating raw meat and food led to diseases, infections, and numerous other health problems. The fire eventually developed into a tool that would fuel inventions, from the gas lamp to coal-powered locomotives.

The very act of using fire for cooking developed humans further. It made us increasingly curious about our surroundings. It is not wrong to say that cooking made humans smarter. Who would have thought?

Think of the connection between water and fire: water created life, and fire helped sustain it. Isn't that wonderful? But there's more.

When ancient Chinese philosophers studied nature and its complexities, they began to observe various details that gave them profound insights into life.

One of the features they focused on was the rising of the sun. Each morning, the sun would gradually illuminate the landscape around them.

This illumination allowed them to enjoy the majesty of the land and all that it held. It also allowed them to wander around, searching for life, food, and objects. However, during sunrise, only one side of the mountain could enjoy the light. The other side was still shrouded in darkness.

The side that was revealed in all its glory by the light was called yang. The side covered in darkness was called yin.

Each morning, yang brought life. It supported the growth of trees, plants, and flowers. It helped people see clearly, allowing them to transport goods, fish, and carry out daily life.

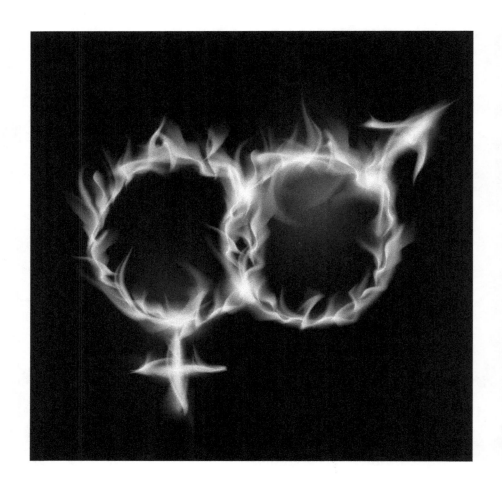

The warmth from the sun could be felt on the skin. Certain flowers even turned toward its rays.

At the same time, the other side of the mountain was covered in darkness. Nature could not enjoy the gift of sunlight. Bandits would often use the darkness to hide in the woods.

Other creatures that preferred the dark would move about until the sunlight would eventually reach them.

Heat and passion were on the yang side, while there was a sense of coldness and alienation on the yin.

However, that distinction would be temporary.

Eventually, when the sun was at its peak, it would illuminate both the yang and yin. And, when it was approaching sunset, only the yin side would be illuminated while yang became shrouded in darkness. This way, yin becomes yang, and yang is turned into the yin.

Now, let's look at how most modern philosophies hold the concept of gender. When people think men and women are different, like two sides of a coin, they continue to remain different.

Heads do not become tails, and neither does the tails side shift position. Each side remains as it is. This philosophy prevents the two genders from even attempting to discover common ground.

Time to shift focus. Let's examine the roles and characteristics of men and women using yin and yang. Now you might ask yourself, which gender is yin and which is yang?

The simple answer is neither – both genders are yin and yang. Allow us to explain. You see, the concept of yin and yang shows that anything that has light is also capable of having darkness.

If you apply that concept to men and women, it is akin to saying that both genders have positive aspects, and both have negative ones. Men and women are both capable of showing kindness, love, compassion, and other positive traits.

They are equally capable of hate, causing pain, and other displays of negative characteristics. Neither gender is perfect. When you understand gender through such a unique perspective, you realize that some pre-established ideas don't hold so much weight anymore.

Traditionally, men were supposed to be the doers. They were expected to be stoic and often aggressive. Women, on the other hand, were the housekeepers. They were less assertive and typically demure.

But with the philosophy of yin and yang, the traditional rules and principles have been turned on their heads. No longer are women confined to the household. They can be aggressive and achieve what they want in life.

At the same time, men don't have to hide their emotions or be afraid of staying at home and taking care of the children while the women work. Sure, some of these concepts might still be rather alien in some parts of the world, but the lines don't exist when it comes to yin and yang.

Men and women both can be determined, confident, supportive, emotional, and loving.

Let's look at the word 'alpha' as an example. Some people believe that alpha is a sexist term that reeks of misogyny.

However, when you examine the animal kingdom – particularly the wolf, since the term alpha is usually attributed to a pack leader – then you are bound to notice that the alpha is a genderless term.

There is both an alpha male wolf and an alpha female. Both live in perfect harmony. It has been said that when one wolf dies, the partner dies of starvation as it refuses to eat in the absence of its mate.

And that union is exactly what is expressed in Tantra. A joining of the sexes. An eradication of borders and stereotypes. It abolishes men's and women's traditional roles, placing them on the same level to examine relationships from a balanced perspective.

The Sexual Energy

When you consider that the male and female forms are given equal reverence, you realize that both men and women can harness the same sexual energy within them.

However, when talking about sexual energy, it seems that we once again find ourselves in the form of thinking that does not fully understand the scope of sex. Many people try to alienate sexual energy.

They feel that there are two forms of energy: one that is sexual and another that includes everything else, from emotional to physical energy. But there is a better way to think of these energies – and to do that. We need to look into physics.

—

According to the first law of thermodynamics, commonly known as the Law of Conservation of Energy, it is accepted among the scientific community that energy cannot be created or destroyed. It can only be changed or transferred from one form to another.

This concept of energy is also applied to Tantra. You see, one cannot create a separate type of energy called sexual energy. All forms of energy are the same; they merely shift from one form to another and back again if required. They are a vital component of your life force, and they are rather fluid, flitting back and forth through various actions, emotions, and even expressions.

Whether you express energy through athletics, music, or art, it is the same energy. Your emotional and physical beings also utilize the same energy. Think that is impossible?

Think about a time when you were so busy at work that by the end of the day, the only thing you could think about was a hot shower, a wonderful meal, and the feeling of those soft pillows beneath your head.

Yet as soon as you reached home, you realized that your favorite sport or movie was on TV. Or perhaps your friends called to meet up for a drink, or you felt the urge to play your

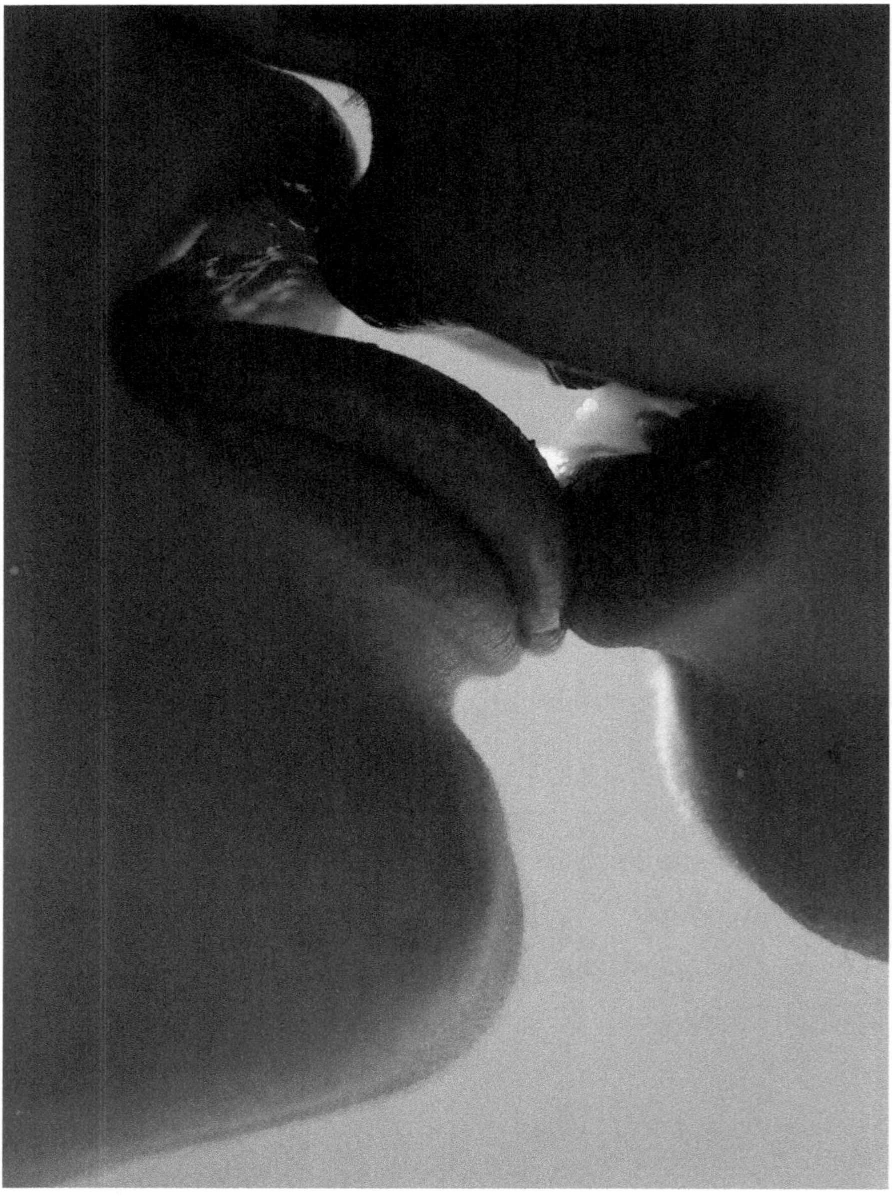

favorite video game, and you decided to postpone sleep for a little while. So what happened? Weren't you too physically exhausted to do anything? How is it that you have a sudden burst of energy to keep going for another activity?

The answer to those questions is that earlier, your emotional and physical energies were low. But once you gained a little boost of emotional energy as you thought of the activity you would like to do, you gained a similar boost to your physical energy levels.

This connection between the physical and emotional or mental states is widely accepted in psychology, as well. For example, poor physical health can increase the likelihood of a person developing mental health problems. Simultaneously, poor mental health can affect one's physical well-being (Mental Health Foundation, n.d.).

As such, the energies that we use for our emotions and physical aspects are the same.

Sexual energy is drawn from the same energy pool shared by emotional and physical states. In sex, we use physical acts to reach new heights of pleasure and the emotional capacity to feel joy, bliss, excitement, and peace.

This understanding of the energies within us allows Tantra to provide us with the means to enhance our lives physically, emotionally, and spiritually.

Sex, Love and All the Good Stuff

When you understand how connected sex is to the mind and body, you begin to realize how much influence it has on love. For this reason, many couples often feel that the 'magic' in the relationship has gone when they discover that their sex life does not hold the same excitement it used to.

We often tend to feel that sex and love are no longer satisfactory. Sex itself loses its erotic, orgasmic, fun, lively, romantic, and spiritual characteristics.

It becomes a force capable of harnessing physical energies but incapable of tapping into the emotional energies that make it special. It begins to lose its level of fulfillment.

In other words, sex becomes similar to washing the dishes or going to work; there is nothing special about it anymore. This leads to sexual problems characterized by frigidity, impotence, faked orgasms, premature ejaculations, sexual disinterest, and ambivalence.

All of these factors are harmful to any relationship, not only because they diminish the value of the relationship but also cause substantial emotional strains on the couple. Pretty soon, these emotional pressures begin to affect other life areas, such as relaxation, work, chores, and even parenthood in many cases.

So, how does Tantra analyze this?

Through a lens of intelligence.

One of the best aspects of Tantra is how it examines ideas and concepts from an intelligent perspective. It does not simply accept anything that is preached by cultures or religions. It seeks first to analyze them and, if they are positive influences, incorporate them into its tradition.

Similarly, we need to begin examining sex from a unique perspective.

The first thing to realize is that sex is also an act of mindfulness. It brings you to the present, allowing you to feel at peace. You forget the troubles of the past and the challenges of the future.

All that matters are how you feel in the here and now. It is food for the spirit, a physical dance that brings orgasmic ecstasy to mind.

Tantra also believes that sex involves a divine element. Sadly, not many people think of sex that way. Why? Because they do not know how to hold intelligent conversations about it. Sex is often related to reproduction.

Think about it – the works on sex and reproduction are numerous. After all, it is a biological process. However, the concept of sex and divinity is minimal. Who wants to think of sex in such a manner?

Chapter 4.
Main Benefits of Tantric Sex

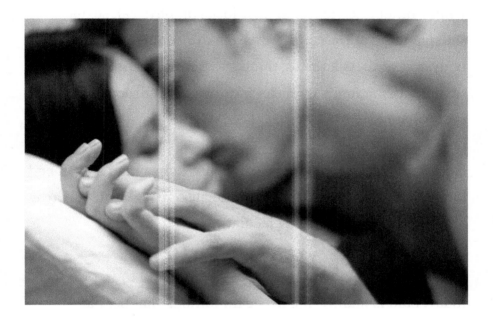

Tantra has been used for thousands of years to make people happy in life. Which includes sexual satisfaction. With Tantric sexual advice, it is possible for every man to give his partner breathtaking orgasms and long-lasting orgasms and with an increased level of sexual pleasure.

Indeed, Tantric sexual advice generally leads a man to a new approach to sex with great amazing achievements and great satisfaction. Below are some benefits of Tantric advice for sex.

Tantra is about supporting and stimulating the innate sensual spirituality of a man. By applying these principles, one can enter a new area of sexual awareness by discovering parts of himself that were previously oppressed.

Unlike other sex tricks that only focus on physical, sexual satisfaction, Tantra emphasizes a man's connection with his body and soul. As a result, thanks to Tantric techniques of sexual satisfaction, a man can improve his bedroom's artificial performance.

Said artificial consciousness would also help a man stay in bed longer and thus make Tantric artificial counseling an effective tool to prevent premature ejaculation.

Sexual freedom is something that most men in the world miss today. Said is mainly due to the inhibitions that people develop as they age.

It is also because of the many unresolved fears and emotional problems that men have in the bedroom. It is, therefore, not surprising that several people have problems in their sex lives.

This is one of the main reasons for the lack of sexual satisfaction in the bedroom, simply because people have erectile dysfunction and other conditions such as premature ejaculation.

Tantra's meditative approach has long been refined to ensure that people, named men, can enjoy sharing and enjoying themselves, especially sex.

Tantra embraces sex as a friend and does not consider it a necessary evil, as some people do. It is believed that sex is a gift from nature and must be valued and explored beyond its unlimited limits.

We learn that sex is perfect, on the condition that his mind, soul, and body go together with that of her partner. Said in general, improved the degree of intimacy between couples and therefore set the stage for great orgasms and artificial satisfaction.

With increased sexual awareness and sexual freedom, Tantric artificial techniques' application allows the free flow of universal and artificial energy between couples. Tantra usually ensures deeper levels of intimacy. Thus, great sexual performance.

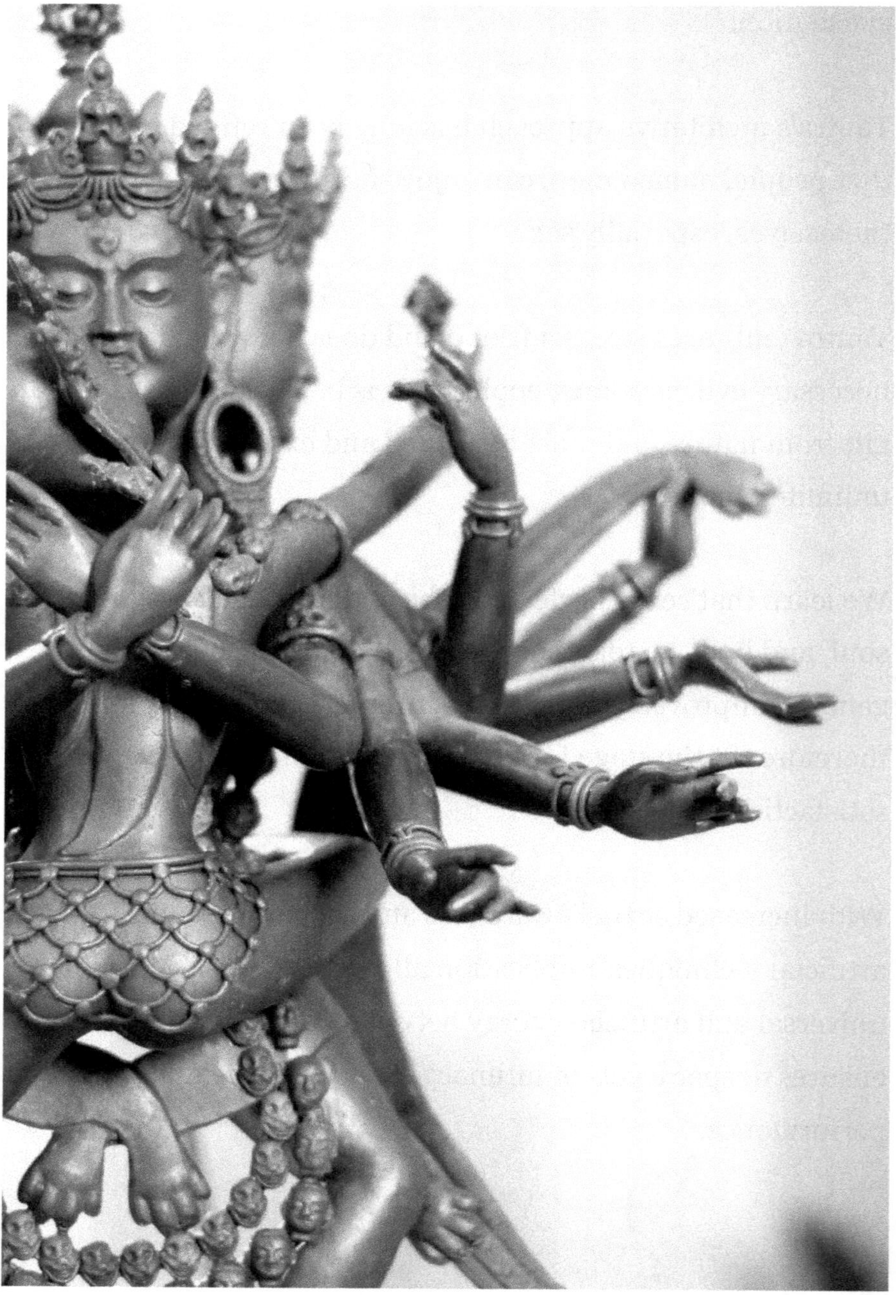

Benefits of Tantric Sex

The benefits of practicing Tantric sex are many. Tantric sex states have long been associated with theta wave states similar to those obtained through meditation.

The primary purpose of these high states of sexual energy was to achieve unity consciousness with life. Any sexual activity is not only beneficial for the body but also to the psyche.

We know that when we are in a state of high sexual arousal, the body releases hormones that give us a sense of euphoria and flood the endocrine system.

Sexual energy nourishes our body and gives us a sense of vitality. By making love, we open our hearts to each other, and we allow ourselves to receive and please.

Sacred sexuality goes beyond that to teach us the deeper inner realms of our psyche and provide us with true understanding and compassion.

With passionate and sensual awareness, you can improve the quality of your sex life.

By practicing Tantric sex, you can awaken what is called "Kundalini" energy.

This energy is very beneficial for you. Tantric sex allows you to understand the power of this sexual energy. Sexual energy is one of the most powerful energies on the planet.

When it is cultivated in the body, it can bring you into an ecstatic state of being and your physical and emotional state of being healed.

An expert in the field of extended orgasm explains that when a person is in an orgasm for a long period, he can process his emotional state much more easily and, at the same time, receive pleasure.

It is a very different way to see emotional compensation and much more pleasure.

The Tantric school of thought now used in the West is called Neo-Tantra.

It combines white (devotional) and red Tantra (sexual) with Yoga and meditation principles. It weaves both sensuality and spirituality so that the practitioner regards the act of making love as sacred.

A loose tradition, to begin with, the Tantric teachings offer no definite trace of their origins. Some believe they started using bodily fluids as a sacrifice to the Tantric deities.

Even the definition of the word "Tantra" is varied and is sometimes defined as "web," "weaving," "expansion," and "liberation." Whatever the definition, the heart of Tantra includes honest communication, creating intimacy, and self-realization.

Self-realization is infinite and goes beyond space and time. The Hindu-Buddhist Tantra's ultimate goal is self-realization, leading to complete peace of mind, satisfaction, and awareness of unity.

It does not require that you change your spiritual beliefs for the process to work. Neo-Tantra can also include access to elevated states of consciousness as the primary goal.

But for most Western practitioners, this offers another way to enrich, expand, and improve their love. Osho, the "father" of neo-Tantra, said: "The first part must be sex. The second part must be love. The third part must be prayer.

And the fourth must be transcendence. To the subtle, you move. And in the fourth, there must eliminate sex, including

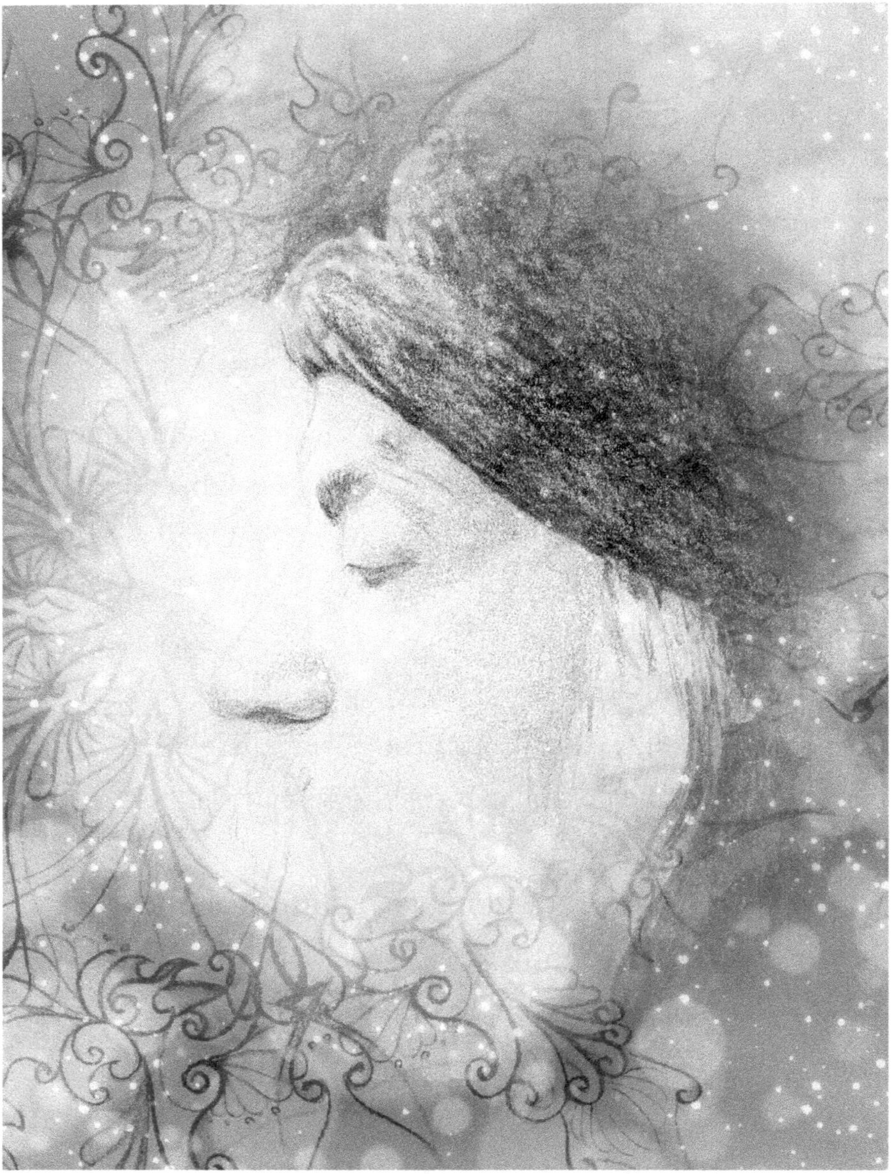

love and prayer, making it absolutely silent, peaceful, and meditative. There is no trace left.

Many unhappy or even frigid women could have a much more satisfying and satisfying life if their loved ones or partners knew how to take care of themselves and their sexual health.

One of the goals of Tantric sex is to cope with this accident and turn it into a positive state of mind using the body's resources.

For many people who are too tired or overly stressed by worries and problems, they are generally somewhat discouraged by life in general and, in particular, are not in the mood to have sex. Unhappy people can also suffer from more diseases than happy people.

Tantric Sex Has Brought a lot of Pleasure

Many women are interested in Tantric sex because of the improvements in sexual health that can be influenced by the stresses and strains of modern life and the stressful lifestyle that many lead today.

Meanwhile, men love Tantric sex because it also focuses on improving erection and ejaculation. Which men won't be interested? Tantric sex is not just your usual "in-out- shaking it all over," and thank you sexual experience.

One of the goals of Tantric sex is to stimulate the endocrine glands to produce more HGH (Human Growth Hormone), serotonin, DHEA, and testosterone.

These hormones help improve sexual health, promote blood circulation in the body, eliminate waste products (toxins, that is), and strengthen the nervous and immune systems to improve overall health.

A person who likes Tantric sex feels healthy and rejuvenated without using any resources or aids. Sex is enough to cause these changes in a person.

However, one must know how to have sex and what to do in bed to achieve this health condition. "

This can be a wonderful self-fulfilling prophecy - improving sexual health and sexual performance also leads to a massive increase in self-esteem and self-confidence, which reinforces a continuous pattern of performance. Successful, better sexual health and confidence, higher self-image.

A man who can regularly give himself and her partner an intense orgasm is happy and healthy. Not to mention that his partner must also have a positive outlook on life and a general feeling of a healthy life.

Tantric sex practitioners claim it has a wonderfully rejuvenating effect on men and women, thereby improving their sexual health.

Frequent and powerful orgasms are a sure way to change a person's mood and relieve anxiety and depression. All diseases that affect the modern mind (such as stress, depression, lack of confidence, and self-respect) can be cured by having sex more often and having better orgasms.

Sexual Secrets That Will Help You Get the Most Out of Tantric Sex

Be in the Rightful Moment:

Most people don't know what's going on with them right now. Be there for fun.

Make sure you have the Right Circumstances:

switch off the TV, concentrate, rest, and enjoy the wish.

Develop Sexual Awareness:

be playful, considerate, erotic, and get involved in the sensory moment.

Create a Sensual Atmosphere:

use the power of light, the scent of aromatherapy, the magic of incense, and the toning of music.

Attract Natural Aphrodisiacs:

nature is the key, with sensual foods such as oysters, coconut, and juicy fruit.

Open Your Mind:

expectations can kill the moment! Try things that strengthen you, clarify you, and bring you back to the magic of youthful energy.

Release Fears:

inhibitions are useless and block who you want to be. It's time to finish who you are. The more you release your fears, the more excited and deeper you will become through the sexual experience.

Be attuned to your Environment:

Feel every sensation, your breathing, your environment, your sounds, your emotions. Whether you are alone or with a partner, be warned.

Discover the Power of Color:

use color therapy by incorporating colored candles, lingerie, lighting, or fabric to bring color to your environment.

Use Your Chakra Energies:

the chakras are stations along the central axis of your being. Each is a point where energy can be expressed in certain actions, attitudes, and emotions.

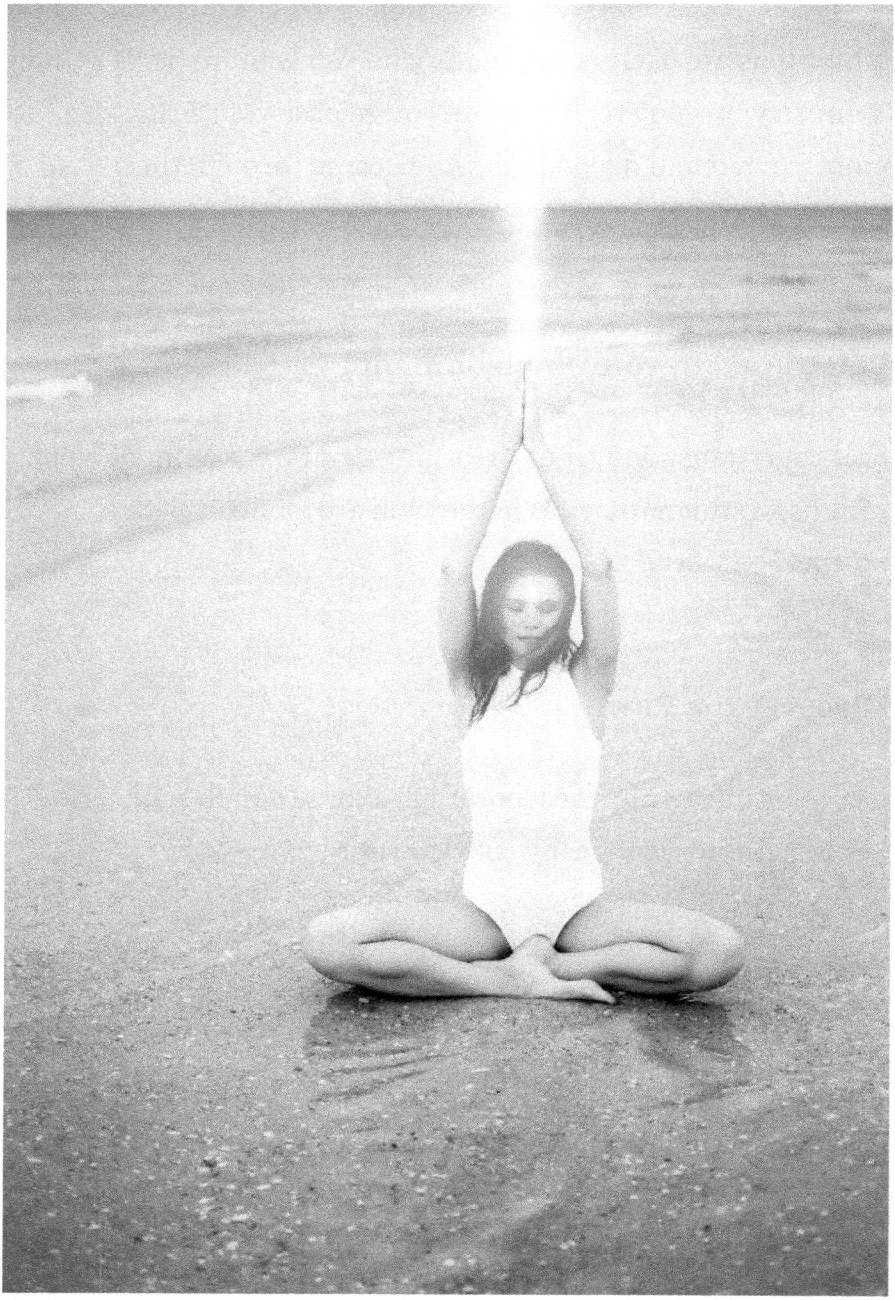

Rev-Up Your Kundalini:

this vital life energy is an ancient system from India that helps the student awaken and merge his spiritual nature.

Give up control:

Powerful mutual concessions. The surrender of power can be just as exciting!

Flow with The Rhythm:

Training is the tendency of two oscillating bodies to lock in phase to vibrate in harmony.

Take your time:

only by exploring the erotic landscape, by enjoying all the hot spots of the body, can we find a way to ultimate fulfillment.

Express your joy:

if it works, let your partner know. Being heard about your pleasure can help seduce your partner. If not, show them where possible.

Liberate or not liberate:

Whether you believe in the great liberation of energy or simply transmute this sexual energy through other channels, there is always pleasure through a Holy Union.

Reaching new heights:

rediscover the deep relationship between sexuality and spirituality.

Sex is the common denominator:

sex is the energetic healer of our mind, body, and spirit.

Honor pleasure as a divine gift:

sex is the most honest aspect of the universal creative life force that electrifies every phase of our lives.

Cultivate Pure ecstasy:

the goal of your Tantric practice is to trigger high states of sexual arousal while remaining completely relaxed.

Chapter 5.
Get in Touch with the Tantric Zone

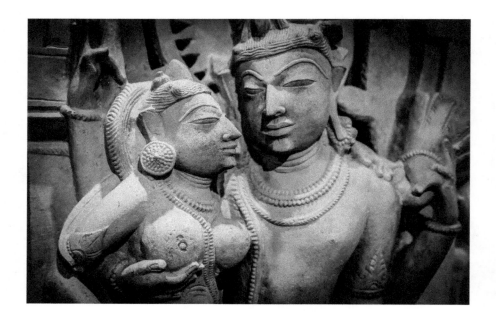

Sensuality is an important part of Tantric sex, and sometimes sensuality can make people uncomfortable.

If you're not used to having sex that focuses on sensuality, the powerful emotions brought out by sensual touching, kissing, and other actions can be a bit overwhelming.

To prepare for the sensuality of Tantric sex, you should try to get in touch with your sensuality before you engage in Tantric sex with a partner. Here are some ways that you can bring out your sensual side:

Take a hot bath – Feel the water's heat and the way the water feels on your skin. Pay attention to the small details like how the cold air feels when you get out of the tub and the roughness of the towel as you dry off.

Buy some silk lingerie – When you are wearing the lingerie, you will automatically feel more sensual but buy some high-quality lingerie and feel the cloth's softness and the way the silk feels on your skin. That will help you feel more sensual.

Engage all your senses – Sensuality doesn't just come from touch. All the senses contribute to sensuality. So, listen to some music that you are passionate about.

Buy some scented candles that have wonderful scents. Surround yourself with things that make you feel sexy and sensuous. Allow yourself to relax and be more aware of your sexuality.

Get a massage – If you are not used to being touched, you can get more comfortable with touch by getting a massage. A hot stone massage is very relaxing and will evoke a different sensual feeling due to the river stones used in the massage.

Getting regular massages will make you more comfortable in your skin and more comfortable being touched.

Bring Out Your Partner's Sensual Side

You can also help your partner bring out their sensual side so that sex is better for both of you. Sensuality and shared energy are the core of Tantric sex, so it will help make the sexual experience more powerful if the two of you engage in a little sensual play together. Here are some ways that you can bring out your partner's sensual side as well as your own:

- Massage – Give your partner a massage that will just get them used to be touched all over their body. Use warm oil to make the massage even more sensual.

- Swim – Go swimming together or bathe together. Playing in the water will allow you to experience new sensations and become more comfortable with intense physical sensations.

- Go to a concert – Music is a very sensual art that can evoke deep passions and feelings. Go to a symphony performance or concert together as a date. Dress up and take a lot of care getting ready, then go and lose yourself in the music. You will both feel more passionate afterward.

- Go to a nice restaurant – Eating can also be a very sensuous experience. Go out for a nice meal together at a restaurant you don't normally go to. The meal doesn't have to be super fancy, but it should be more than a burger at the local family restaurant. Try a new cuisine that neither of you has tried before.

Undress your partner – After a long day, pull your partner aside and slowly undress him or her, taking care to allow them to feel the sensations of the clothing as you remove it. You can also shower or bathe him/her if you want to create a sensuous experience.

Talk About Sex

Communication is important in any relationship, but many couples find it difficult to communicate about sex. Even though sex is the cornerstone of a good relationship, many couples never bother to discuss sex or talk about what feels good to them with their partner.

For Tantric sex to bring you closer together, it's important that you be able to talk about sex openly with your partner and for your partner to be able to talk to you openly too.

If you and your partner have not had a lot of success trying to talk to one another about sex in the past, here are some ideas to open the lines of communication and make it easier to talk about sex together:

- Schedule a time to talk about sex – The time to talk about your sexual desires, fantasies, and preferences isn't when you are sitting down to dinner, or when you are driving the kids to practice, or when you both are exhausted from a long day. Schedule a time to talk when both of you are rested and ready to talk openly with one another. Maybe you can schedule a bath together after the kids are in bed. Or maybe you can arrange a little early morning time before work. Find a time that will lead to a productive conversation and put it on the schedule.

- Use examples to discuss your fantasies or things that you want to try – If there is a book that you read that contains a fantasy scene, you'd like to try to buy your partner a copy and highlight that scene. Alternatively, suggest that you watch a movie that you find sexy together and point out things you'd like to try with your partner. When you can give concrete examples, it can help your partner know exactly what you want to try.

- Be open to new things – When your partner talks to you about their sexual desires, don't judge what they say. Think about it and let it sit for a minute or two so that you can figure out how you feel about it. If it's something that you're not sure about, agree together to discuss it at a different time after you have had some time to think about it. And give your partner the time to consider your desires as well.

Experience New Things Together

A great way to reconnect with your partner and build a better connection between you is to experience new things together sexually.

Tantric sex is all about celebrating sexual energy and raising sexual energy. How you do that is up to you. So, when you and your partner are comfortable discussing your fantasies or things that you would like to try together, the next step is to make some of those fantasies a reality.

Here are some tips to make those new experiences go a little more smoothly:

Keep the lines of communication open – remember that the experience is new for both of you.

You both need to communicate what feels good, what doesn't, and what else you would like your partner to do. Giving and receiving feedback during the experience will help be a fun and pleasant experience for both of you.

- Keep your sense of humor – When you are trying out something new, things will often go awry in strange and sometimes hilarious ways. Look for the humor in the situation and roll with the punches. If an experience is not at all what you both expected it to be or if it falls flat, just laugh it off and focus on each other. No matter what, the experience should stress love and positivity between the two of you.

- Practice first – If your fantasy involves equipment like silk ties, handcuffs, a flogger, or any other type of equipment, practice with that equipment before you try it out on your partner. That way, you can be sure that your partner won't get injured, and you won't end up hurting yourself or breaking something.

Set ground rules – When you talk about your fantasies, you should always discuss your limits and ground rules for any encounter. Making the boundaries clear is the best way to ensure that both of you have a good time and enjoy the experience.

Keep Sex Playful

Even though Tantric sex celebrates the spiritual side of sex, it doesn't have to be super serious or solemn. It's a celebration, and it should be fun.

Sex should be fun. Tantric sex allows couples the freedom to experiment with anything and everything that will raise their sexual energy and give expression to the sacred energy that each person has.

While Tantric sex should never be rushed or hurried, it doesn't have to be hours long grind either. There are plenty of ways that you can enjoy each other in a fun and playful way during Tantric sex like:

- Giving and receiving massages

- Playing erotic board games or party games

- Experimenting with sex toys

- Indulging in some fantasy play

- Taking a bath or a shower together

- Fantasy play

To keep things light, be sure to go slow and enjoy the playtime. Don't only focus on having an orgasm. The more you play, the more sexual energy you will raise. Sexual play is also a great way to connect on a deeper level so that your relationship will be stronger.

Don't Forget to Breathe

One of the most important parts of Tantric sex is breathing. The process of taking slow, meditative breaths while you are engaged in intercourse is part of what makes the experience a sacred sexual experience. Slowing down your breathing and focusing on your breath will heighten your consciousness and raise your sexual energy.

During sex, it's common for people to breathe more rapidly and breathe shallowly because of physical exertion and mental

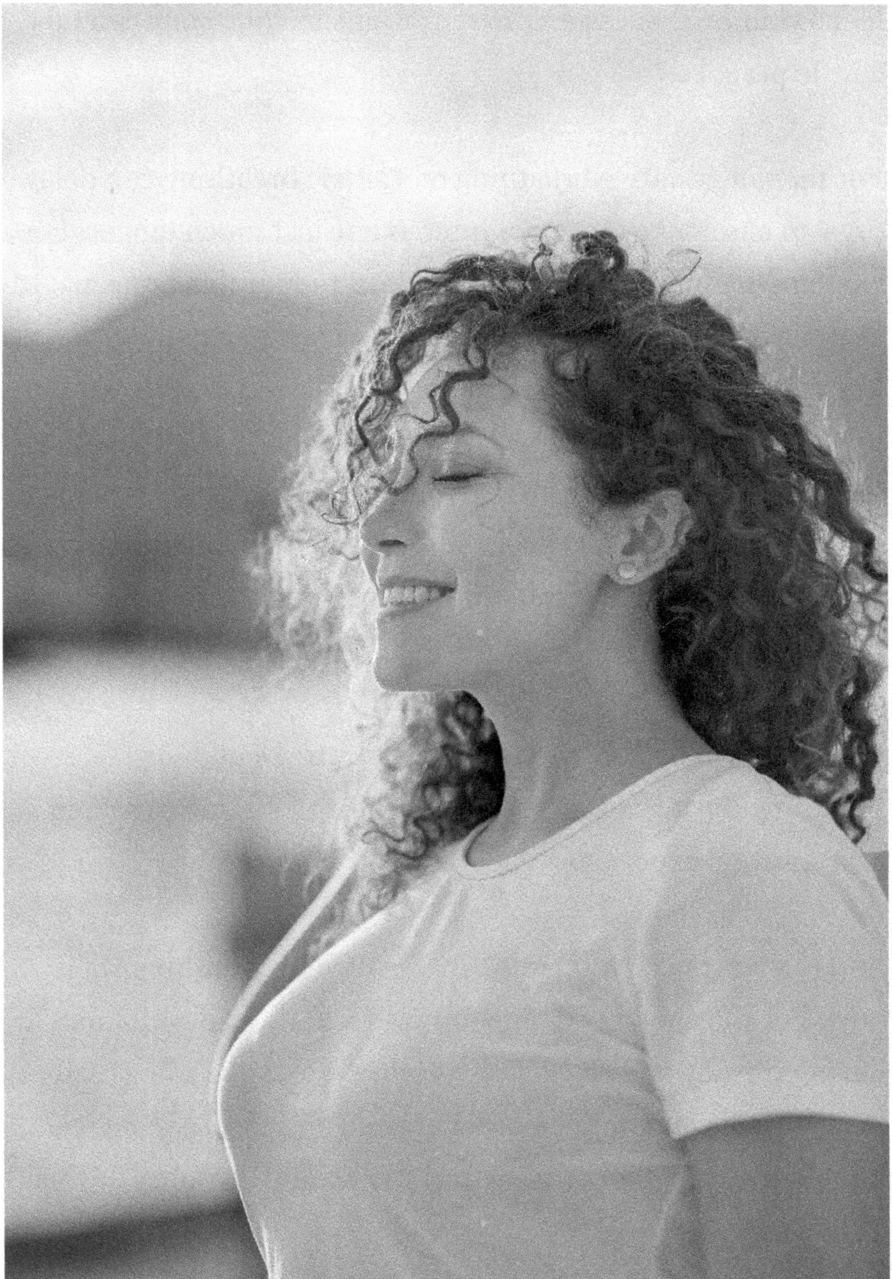

stimulation. So to physically slow your breathing down and focus your awareness on the sensations in your body can take a little practice.

For men, meditative breathing or Tantric breathing can delay orgasm and make the act of intercourse last much longer. For women, meditative breathing can lead to multiple orgasms. It also makes the emotional experience of sex much more intense.

To become good at meditative breathing during sex, it helps to practice meditation at other times. By meditating regularly, you will get better at regulating your breath and focusing your mind.

Then you will be able to use those skills to focus your breathing during sex and change the act of sex into a sacred and spiritual experience.

You can start becoming more aware of your breathing right now. For the next few days, stop yourself at various points during the day and check how you breathe. Take a few really deep breaths and notice how energized and focused you feel. That is the type of breathing that you should be doing during Tantric sex.

When you first start focusing on your breath during sex, it's ok to stop your partner and suggest that both of you focus on your breathing for a few minutes.

Sit opposite from each other and hold hands. Look into each other's eyes and focus on matching your breathing. Try to do that for ten or even twenty minutes. When you return to sexual activity, it will be much more intense.

Soul Gazing

Another important part of Tantric sex is eye contact. Because the eyes are truly the windows to the soul, to make sex a sacred experience, you should use eye contact and other methods to increase the bond and connection you have. Tantric Soul Gazing is one ritual that you can do to bond deeply with your partner.

To perform the Soul Gazing ritual, you should meditate first or practice some meditative breathing. Both of you should be sitting comfortably and facing each other. You can sit in chairs, or on the bed, or cushions on the floor. It doesn't matter as long as you are comfortable. You should be touching in some way.

You can hold hands, or you can each put your hands on the other person's knees. It doesn't matter how you touch. Just make sure that you are touching so that you are forming a closed energy circuit. Close your eyes to practice meditative breathing.

When you are both ready, open your eyes, and make eye contact. Each of you should look at the other person's left eye because the left eye is the most receptive to Eastern traditions. Focus on the other person's left eye and look. See that person's soul reflected in their eyes as they see yours.

You can blink, and you can shift your body if you need to, but don't stop looking into each other's eyes for at least five minutes. The longer you look at each other, the deeper of a connection you will feel.

You can practice the Soul Gazing ritual as foreplay before sex, or you can practice it during sex if you want to make your sexual intercourse a truly sacred event.

Sometimes, people find the Soul Gazing ritual overwhelming at first because they feel very vulnerable, letting someone look so deeply into their soul. If you or your partner feel uncomfortable, go slowly and gradually increase the amount of time you spend maintaining deep eye contact.

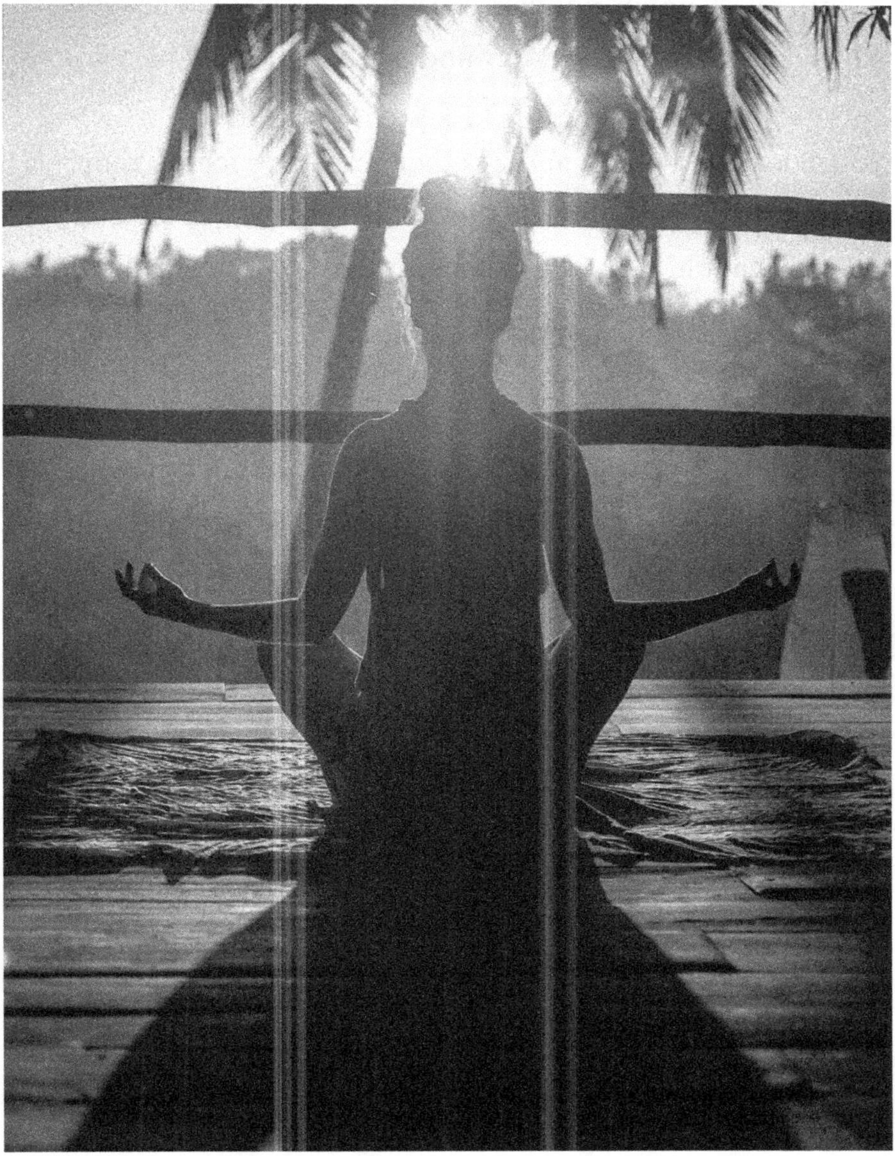

Touch Your Partner

Another very important part of Tantric sex is touching your partner. Touch builds energy and increases sexual pleasure.

Touch is very sensual, and whether you are touching your partner with your hands or a prop like a feather or a piece of silk, you should make sure there is plenty of touching before any actual intercourse occurs.

Massage is an important element of Tantric sex, but not all touching has to be a massage. Here are some fun ways that you and your partner can incorporate touching into you foreplay without giving or receiving massages:

- Undress each other

- Bathe each other

- Feed each other a sensual snack like chocolate-covered strawberries

- Brush your partner's hair

- Caress your partner's entire body over their clothing, and then again with clothing off

- Hug for five minutes or more

- Hold hands

- Lay quietly together with your bodies touching and feel each other

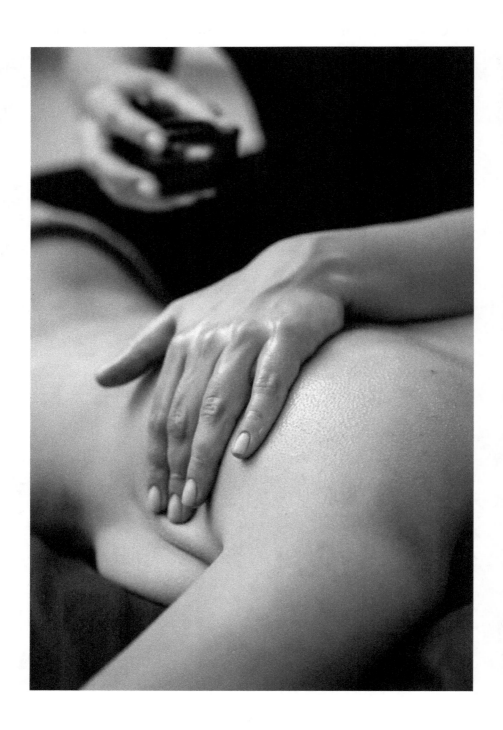

Chapter 6. Tantric Massage

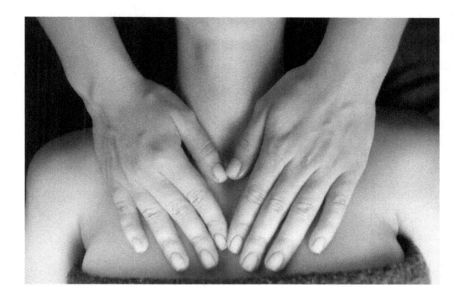

A tantric massage adores touch loaded with consideration and nearness, without a standard structure and foreordained outcome.

Tantra massage is given from the heart. In a tantric massage, the whole body takes part, and sexual zones can also be contacted, consistently with deference for (common) limits. Tantra massage is a fiery massage wherein sexual vitality additionally gets consideration. A tantric massage happens based on fairness and sets up a private association between massage providers and recipients.

Rationally, physically, on a fundamental level, and now and then even at the profundities of a central core. A tantric massage's motivation is to "bring" the recipient toward (the path of) a characteristic, elated condition of being.

The impact is regularly a brilliant physical, mental prosperity. More often than not, the beneficiary is exceptionally loose, brilliantly streaming and winding up well in the heart and higher circles.

First and significant hint: Be prepared

Even though it might appear to be fairly self-evident, our first tip is: it is so significant that you can give a tantric massage from your heart what's more, that you can get the dash of your body, yet besides, your heart being also contacted, that you should almost certainly get physically involved with yourself before you can give or get a cozy, tantric massage.

So if you or your accomplice feel any wavering about affection or closeness, at that point, we certainly suggest doing initial either of the accompanying courses: "Closeness begins with you" and additionally "Living from an Open Heart."

1. Progressively more liberated bit by bit...

During the massage, yet additionally, when you do various massages in an arrangement, you become increasingly free. This is a procedure of clearing bars and pushing limits: (vivaciously).

What was difficult during the primary massage to give up winds simpler in consequent massages. This is an extremely legitimate and regular procedure. The certainty (in the massage supplier) that it is alright makes the unwinding, the opening, and the give up greater, which is beautiful.

Be that as it may, be careful: no sex

Less beautiful is that the giver and beneficiary's dynamic closeness frequently prompts dynamic and (un) attractive sexuality among benefactor and beneficiary. Outskirts change, and it is essential to do this all around deliberately. Oozing sexuality is fine; however, sex and sexual acts centered around joy gratification do not have a place with a tantric massage. It is by no means OK if the provider in a tantric massage forces his own body/sexuality/sexual wants. Tantra massage is focused on the characteristic, blissful condition of being.

2. Think about the desires and wants of the beneficiary

We frequently hear that individuals "take" a tantric massage for a specific reason. Men long for an upbeat consummation; ladies regularly need "recuperating." It is alright if you have wishes and wants, fine. In any case, understand that it can likewise run all around differently.

It is not something like simply having a fast "Yoni (vaginal) massage" and to attempt to utilize tantric massage as a moment mending system.

Realize that things can unfurl differently

Obviously, behind each tantric massage is a longing, an aim, and that is fine. Significantly, the aims and limits are obvious to everybody. Once in a while, be that as it may, it is marginally different from what you had thought. So express your longing (s) and after that, let go of it. Give up and acknowledge everything that comes.

3. Give criticism and reconciliation minutes

Tantra massage is physical. Utilize your faculties, let your body talk. What's more, give criticism, tell how you feel. So previously, during, and after the massage, you convey in a wide range of ways. Perhaps you are at times overpowered by the impact of the massage, however consistently remain intentionally present, continue feeling.

Together, require some investment (during and) after the massage, allow things to sink, give mix minutes. During as well as in the primary days after the massage, numerous things can occur.

A tantric massage can truly relax up everything. Appreciate the massage, and appreciate the radiance. Regardless of whether it is less pleasant, at that point, understand that it is beneficial for you that it fits into your self-awareness process.

4. It is constantly an enthusiastic massage

Enacting and letting free the progression of life vitality (prana) is the tantric massage's principal part. Tantra massage is a vigorous massage wherein sexual vitality additionally gets consideration.

In a tantric massage, the entire body takes part, and erogenous zones can likewise be contacted. This consistently with deference for (common) limits. When enacting life vitality, sexual vitality assumes a significant job. In tantric massage we play with the actuation of essential/sexual/enthusiastic/energetic/love/creation/natural vitality.

Start with the heart

Nothing is compulsory, yet we propose that it is great to begin the real massage with the heart (chakra) soon after the principal attunement. Opening the heart and initiating the heart's vitality is magnificent.

Particularly in men, the heart chakra is regularly (as well) shut. Opening only, it can be a magnificent encounter. It is additionally an incredible beginning for ladies. Heart vitality can be tenderly brought down and bolstered when opening the sex chakra. Additionally, see beneath under the heading "restored parity and association among sex and heart."

5. Try not to release, yet energize

Finding sexuality, sexual incitement, Yoni, or Lingam massage is good, be that as it may, a tantric massage does not actuate sexual vitality to release (joy) yet to energize. To free the sexual vitality, add it to your life vitality and let it stream in your body. It is tied in with spreading neighborhood sexual vitality, changing the sexual vitality, opening the body (the Yoni), and discharging pressure, blockages, and so forth. Furthermore, to carry you into the characteristic state (to charge).

Body climaxes

As the impact of tantric massage approaches the characteristic condition of being, there is less to state about it. What is euphoria? What is an orgasmic body? The best thing is if you experience it yourself.

The truth of the matter is that your body at that point is very vivaciously charged and simultaneously totally loose. In the body climax, there is profound unwinding; a profound give up in which you, your conscience me, vanish totally. You are never again here.

That snapshot of giving up might be longer because of tantric massage. Seconds, minutes, 60 minutes? Who knows.... Your body may stun a little, every one of the cells vibrates in an enjoyably blissful recurrence. You are not there but then again ... Mmm... an orgasmic condition of being.

Heart climax

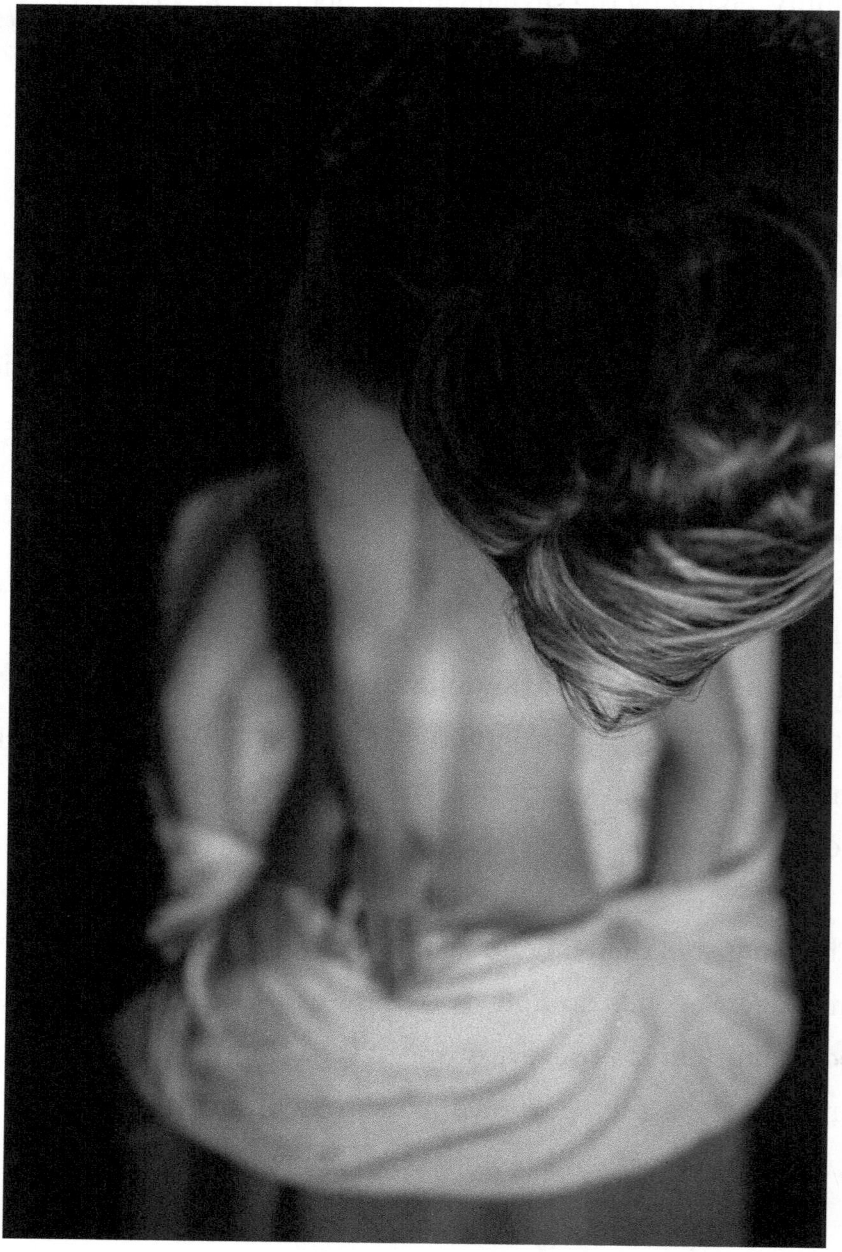

A heart climax can happen if the body is adequately loose and open. If there is a level of giving up that permits the sexual/life vitality to open the heart (totally). It feels like the climax happens in the heart.

This experience is typically exceptionally overpowering. We are not used to living with an open heart. So rely on a great deal of feeling, and do not fear it (both as supplier and beneficiary). It is a pleasant gift to offer and to get.

Start with the heart

The heading is: from sex to the heart (or the other way around). An over-burden of sexual vitality is brought to the heart (stroking). Along these lines, the heart chakra opens more.

Continuously, prana is spread all through the body. Progressively the entire body is opened and fiery or orgasmic. Even though the ordinary sex climax likely could be a piece of tantric massage, the massage is consistently toward holiness, of the normally overjoyed condition of being.

6. Self-esteem and cognizance are significant! '

When initiating and feeling (sexual/enthusiastic) vitality, much mindfulness and love (security) is required. In human life, we (as an infant/tyke/youthful/grown-up) experience numerous circumstances that unequivocally limit our life vitality.

Our vitality framework is, in this way, isolated (sex and heart). A ton of vitality will likewise be put away in our bodies (solidify) when in high sway circumstances, we cannot battle or flight.

Massage triggers

Contacting and discharging both the solidified vitality during the massage (little/major passionate injuries) and the body strain (shield) regularly creates very a few responses. Many people have sexual taboos, damage(s), and molding, and at the sexual level, there are regularly a significant number of "triggers."

Tantra massage is not treatment; it is significant that both provider and collector are very much aware of this. An excess of vitality, and releasing it too rapidly, is not wise—cognizance (great perception) and cherishing attunement guarantee a decent result.

7. Regard limits

We knew it for quite a while, obviously, however, since the #Me-too disclosures, a few things have come up in the realm of tantric massage. Masseurs (you do not hear a great deal about masseuses) enjoy their very own sexual fulfillment on "customers."

That has close to nothing or nothing to do with tantric massage. The security of both the recipient and the provider should consistently be ensured. Cherishing attunement consistently starts things out.

Clarify understandings ahead of time

Each individual (except for when you are illuminated) has his points of confinement. This is human and is additionally vital. Likewise, read the article on guarding limits). So think in advance, both the provider and the collector, what your cutoff points are. Permit a decent admission and planning, likewise with your darling/massage accomplice.

Clarify understandings ahead of time: about mental limits, clarify physical limits. It is a misguided judgment that a tantric massage should consistently be stripped, rubbish. With garments on is additionally very alright, however, it is difficult to work with (hot) oil. It is likewise a misinterpretation that with a tantric massage, the emphasis ought to be on aligned sexual pieces of the body, for example, bosoms and sex, additionally babble. By and by, we have given and gotten numerous tantric massages on simply just the head. Each cell is sexy, revealed, you will be astonished.

8. Be cognizant to restored solidifying minutes

It frequently goes "wrong" in tantric massage is the point at which a recap of solidified minutes emerges. Old injuries are activated and remembered, without the fundamental self-esteem and attention to appropriately manage it now.

What happens frequently is that the recipient solidifies (never again responds) again, whereby the supplier is not adequately adjusted (present) to see this.

Keep limits from being surpassed once more

The enactment at that point, for the most part, goes excessively far/excessively long, where there is a risk that the (same) limits will be surpassed once more. Both providers and recipients must be exceptionally mindful of this. It stresses the requirement for good correspondence, clear understandings

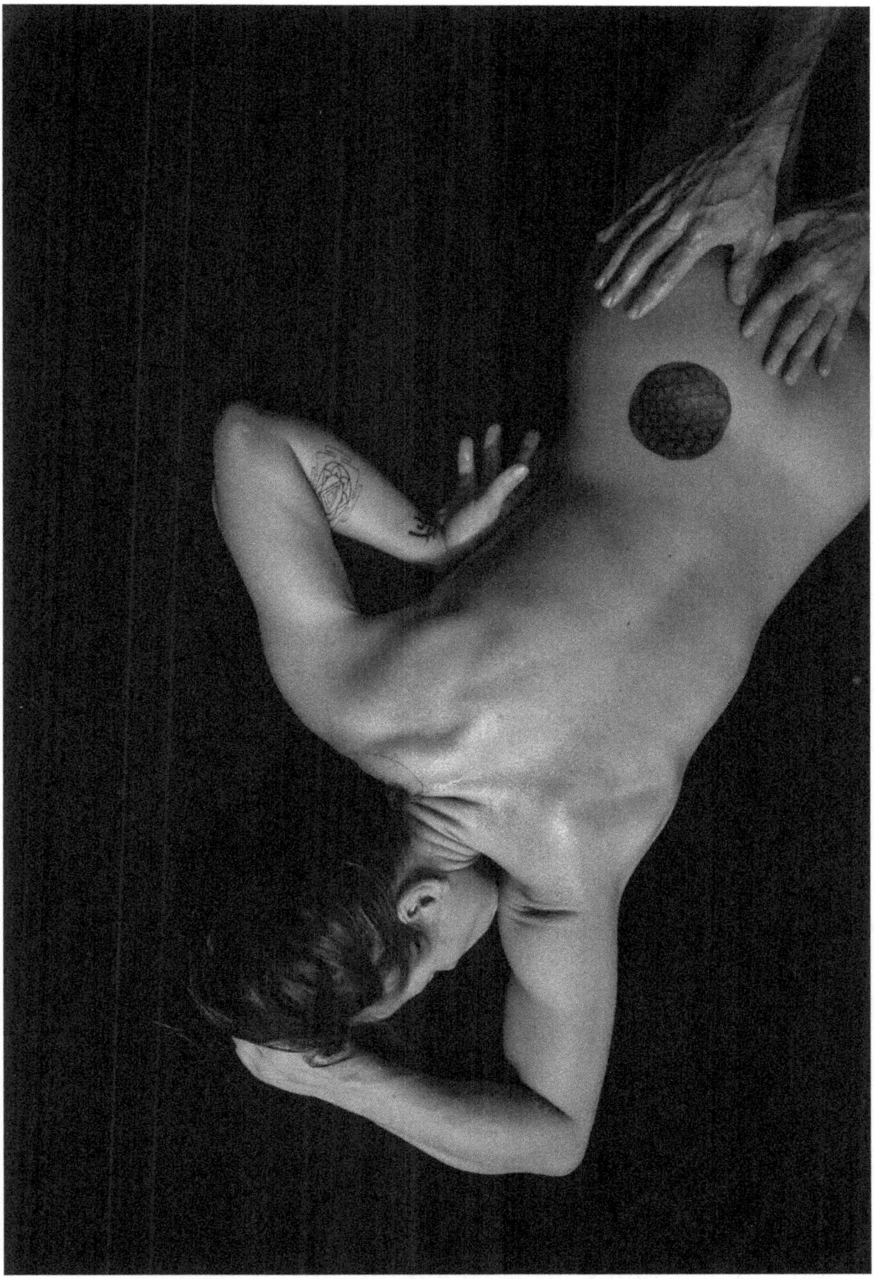

about the limits indeed. Yet, besides, the requirement for adequate input and coordination minutes during the massage.

9. Try not to move in the direction of a specific objective

A tantric massage is constantly different. No one can tell how it goes. It is not the system, or the ideal request of kneading that is significant; it is about what is proper/important. What does the collector most need right now? What is beneficial for her/him?

Love comprehends what to do; love consistently has a proper reaction. Thus, the massage will actually be that which is required. It is adequate that the provider is available and continues checking out his/her heart to the frequencies of adoration.

The awesome additionally has his/her arrangement; you cannot envision that. Tantric massages, in this manner, frequently have an amazing course. Everything fits into a bigger entirety. For instance, a tantric massage does not generally need to be "fine," finishing with ecstasy. A "fizzled" massage can be the initial phase in an extraordinary improvement.

10. Careful discipline brings about promising results

You cannot generally do a tantric massage. Each adoring touch with consideration and nearness is great! Rest guaranteed you do not need to do long stretches of preparing.

You will see that as you get some more experience, you will turn out to be increasingly delicate, both as a provider and recipient. The specialty of contacting... Various components help to bring somebody (quicker/simpler) into that regular (euphoric) condition of being. The level of unwinding, for instance, is one of them. The other? You are certainly going to find them.

11. Request free

A few masseurs are essentially worried about what they find lovely, fun, alluring. Extreme as a supplier you additionally can appreciate; however, the pith is that you are there for the beneficiary.

So disregard your own "needs," avoid your issues, or rather all ... make an effort not to force anything. Nothing must be done; nothing is required! Try not to attempt to constrain anything. Once more, do whatever it takes not to force anything (your very own objectives/body/sexuality)! Check out what the recipient needs. It is for what it is worth, and it keeps running as it goes. Trust in affection. Maybe you are baffled when

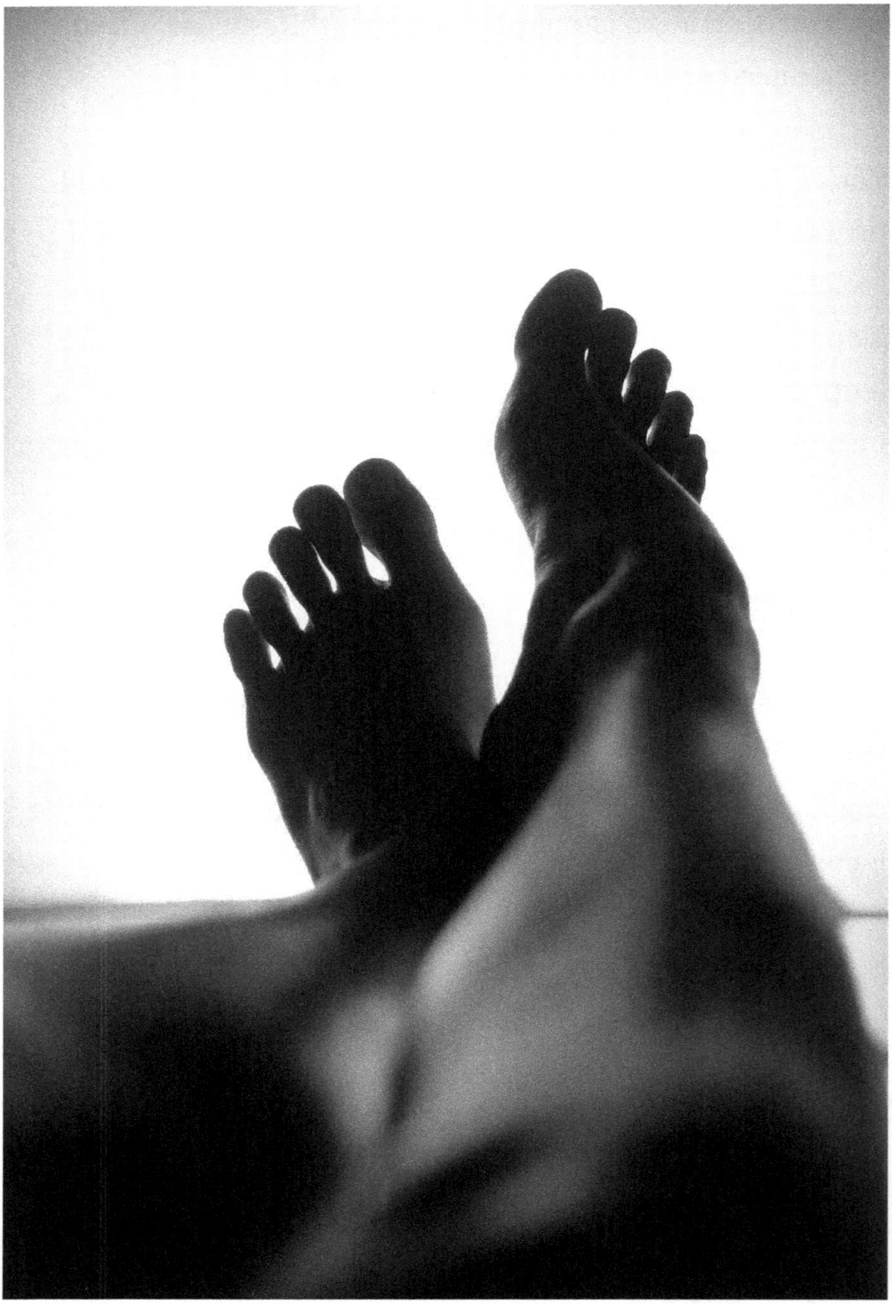

somebody nods off. You may not be hanging tight for a passionate cry, yet a tantric massage has no objective. No proposed outcome. What will be. Acknowledge that.

12. Reestablished parity and association among sex and heart

Actuating sexual (and other) vitality in the chakras is one, parity and stream in the body is two.

The upward and descending stream in our body is frequently coagulated. Particularly the association between sex and heart is aggravated; it happens to nearly everybody during the (pre-) youthful stage. It is very difficult to be open and streaming both in the sex chakra and the heart chakra.

13. Tantra massage is more than sexual fulfillment

Tantra massage has, as we would see it, almost nothing to do with sex. Those searching for sex better can go for (tantric) sex. The individuals who are searching for sexual fulfillment, for an orgasmic discharge (glad consummation) better go for a suggestive massage. To the extent we are concerned, (oral) sex and activities that are only planned for "Cumming" are not part of a tantric massage.

Yoni or Lingam massage

The entire body can take an interest in a tantric massage, including the personal parts. In tantric, the vagina is called Yoni; the penis is called Lingam. Furthermore, they can arrive share in the massage. These two names affirm the exceptional character of what tantric goes for to the extent we are concerned.

The massage sees everything in the world as "divine," as hallowed. Thus we additionally observe the private parts. Bosoms are holy and an association with the heart. The Yoni is a beautiful, consecrated piece of the female body. The Lingam is a ground-breaking, divine piece of the manly.

At the point when the Yoni or Lingam is massaged, they might be seen and respected just because. All taboos fall away, all agony and (butt-centric) pressure (in the end) vanishes. It is decisively the private parts that are places where (misuse) injuries are put away, and much-stifled vitality is available.

Chapter 7. Most Important Benefits of Tantric Massage

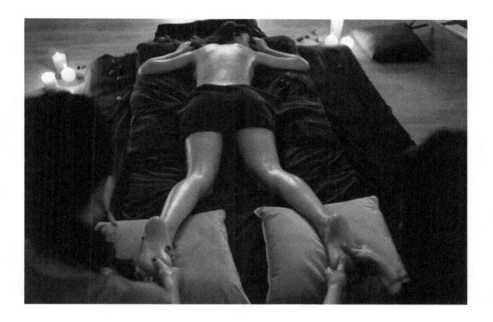

Tantra, and all of its beliefs, have been practiced for over 9,000 years. Way back in the Himalayan Mountains in India, religious leaders fully believed that sexual ritual and fulfilling the sexual aspect of the human form were the ultimate path to a higher form of liberation and connection with the energies of the spiritual world.

In today's world, Tantra's teachings are taken and translated into a full-body experience that doesn't just hinge on the fulfillment of sexual desires and wishes. This traditional message is subsequently heightened by utilizing breathing exercises and genital stimulation (neither of which were used in the olden days).

Not only is the massage benefiting in a relaxing manner, but it can also bring about ways to cope with sexual trauma by slowly tackling the PTSD of the event in a mild, trusting, and controlled environment.

A tantric massage relaxes every single part of the body. It doesn't just address an aching back and stiff shoulders. It tackles every single muscle in the body.

The massage consists of two to three hours of massaging every muscle, both big and small, to release that deep-seated stress that sits in the body's small crevices. This relaxation doesn't just become physical.

It ends up manifesting in a spiritual manner that relaxes the soul as well. After all, 80% of people who experience a tantric massage for the first time end up returning customers.

Not only does a tantric massage revolve around relaxation, but there are also specific breathing techniques that the client is talked through during the massage. These breathing techniques help center the mind, calm the soul, and promote inward reflection and self-awareness.

For those who are slowly overcoming sexual trauma, these breathing techniques are used to slow down the natural adrenal response from PTSD-driven emotions and memories and give them a viable method for self-calming their body during the massage.

The breathing enhances the overall experience and controls those who feel that they have lost it.

A tantric massage can provide a state of emotional healing, as well. It isn't just the physical attributes of the massage that encourage people to come back.

It is also a healthy emotional promotion that draws them back as well. Learning to lean back and receive that kind of pleasure with absolutely no reciprocation contest is a revalidation of self-worth.

This can impact the overall state of happiness of the client, and it can slowly help teach someone that receiving this type of "gift" (as in receiving the "gift" of relaxation and happiness) does not have to come with the stress of having to reciprocate it. It teaches people to slowly accept the happiness that is due

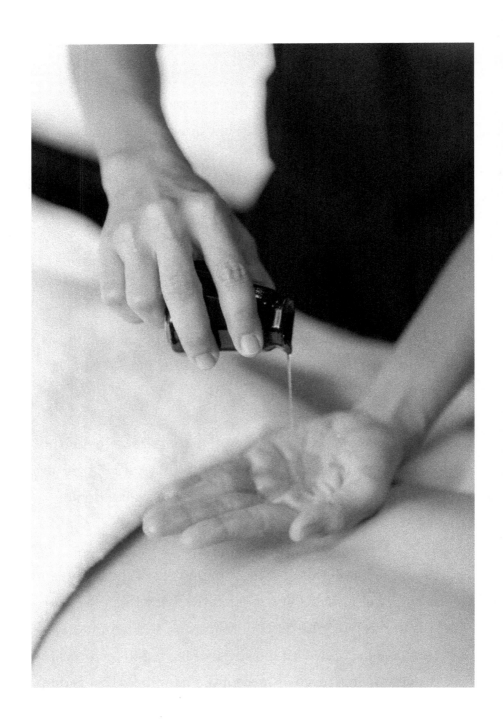

to them without creating imaginary stressors based on how they will be perceived if the actions aren't reciprocated.

However, the pleasurable aspect can't be overlooked. The sheer enjoyment that comes from feeling every single muscle in your body relaxing can be positively overwhelming, and the thrill of the emotional and spiritual balance can become intoxicating.

The physical pleasure is sometimes brought with tantric massages (in the form of orgasm) that can bring on a heightened sense of relaxation and happiness. Keep in mind, however, that orgasm is not the ultimate goal. It never is with a tantric massage.

The spiritual, emotional, and physical relaxation and binding of your energies with the universe are the ultimate goals.

A tantric massage can also help people to curb impulses. The breathing techniques taught and acquired during tantric massages can also be utilized to control other aspects of the client's life, such as food cravings and premature ejaculation.

These natural human impulses can be controlled, just like in the tantric massage, because the breathing techniques promote the re-focusing of one's mind.

And, as if that isn't enough, the mere intensity of the massage and the attention that each of your muscles obtains, the promotion of blood circulation can contribute to many blatant health benefits.

Color can return to the skin, organs can begin to function more efficiently, things such as eyesight and hearing can become better, and even chronic headaches can be treated with better blood circulation that a tantric massage can provide.

A tantric massage can provide a massive amount of benefits. Not only does it have individual benefits that many massages don't tackle, but it also tackles the original benefits of the massage in the first place!

Things such as pain management with extreme muscle tension and fatigue are addressed with the total body attention that a tantric massage can provide. The elongated average time of the massage ensures that every ache and pain that the client is experiencing is fully and completely taken care of.

Also, many people who seek out regular massages to treat migraines and headaches will find the same type of treatments within a tantric massage. Moreover, because a tantric massage promotes the massaging of every muscle in the body, better

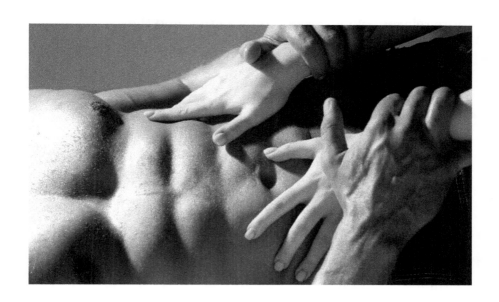

blood circulation can occur long after the client has left the appointment, which means that the massage's effects last longer than that of a regular massage.

However, one of the best benefits that are chronically raved about is the sleep improvements that tantric massages spawn.

The overall quality of sleep is improved because the body is more relaxed, blood circulation is better, and the pain management that a tantric massage can work its way into how your body seeks out sleep, providing an uninterrupted as well as a deeper state of sleep.

The wonderful thing is that absolutely everyone can benefit from a tantric massage. Practicing and learning about Tantra can open up so many different doorways that lead to both an increase in sexual healing and desire and promote a state of self-awareness that not many ever achieve within their lifetime.

The health benefits are overwhelming, and many have professed that they prefer it to medicinal treatments of certain health issues (such as general aches, pains, and headaches). A tantric massage can open up someone's mind and soul to an immense connection between the energies of the world and the physical energies raging within their bodies. It can create an overwhelming sensation that roots them to the ground promotes an overall positive state of mind.

Tantric massage has also been finding its way into the medicinal world. While it isn't a conclusive treatment for anything, the benefits that have been proven can also be rooted in other health issues.

For example, the promotion of better blood circulation can lead to aiding in treating inflammatory diseases. The promotion of self-awareness and breathing exercises can calm and slow down the mind, which can aid people who have been diagnosed with anxiety disorders and A.D.H.D.

With the promotion of relaxation and the reduction of stress that comes with a tantric massage, benefits such as aiding in digestion and hormone imbalances can also be tackled within a few sessions.

While a doctor will never prescribe one for you, the benefits that have been proven with regular massages translate in a deeper aspect to tantric massages, which is why so many people can proclaim so many different benefits.

Tantra proclaims that it can aid in all of these mental and physical disabilities because a tantric massage can relieve energy blockages and readdress energy imbalances within the body. During a tantric massage, the belief is that there are only two things that cause physical pain within the body: a blockage of the flow of blood and the blockage of the flow of energy.

Tantra focuses on promoting better blood circulation through deep breathing and meditation. It focuses on relieving energy blockages through relaxation, circular massaging, and strict attention to every part of the body.

With a tantric massage, no part of the body is neglected (unlike a regular massage, which promotes relaxation and physical purity), and every atom of the client's body is addressed in much the same way. This promotes a physical cohesiveness that translates into a spiritual cohesiveness that is promoted within.

While there is a sexual energy focus, the point is that this is not the main component of a tantric massage. The sexual energy addressed within a tantric massage does not have an end goal of sexual pleasure.

The point is that sexual energy is released within the body, aids in energetic circulation by relieving guilt-ridden and stressed blockages throughout the body, and encourages (via the breathing techniques) to push that energy up through the

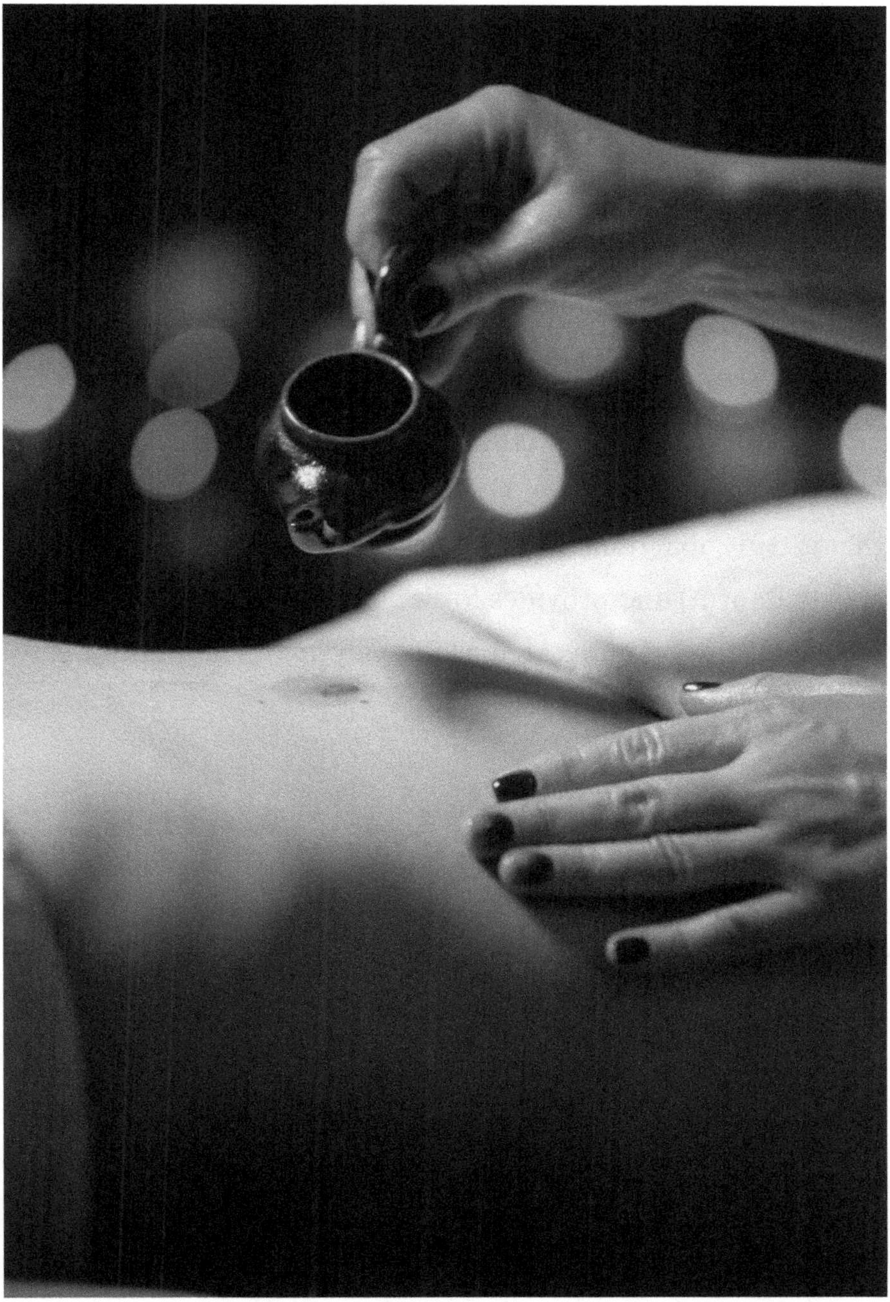

spine so that it can be distributed, filling every cell throughout the entire body. The sexual energy harnessed is not one that seeks a temporary release but seeks a permanent fulfillment of something deeper than the physical body craves.

In Tantra, it is necessary to address all aspects of the basic human form. Those areas are innate needs, such as food, water, movement, and sex.

This does not mean that tantric (and its tantric massages) address every form. It merely means that it focuses on a form that is truly abandoned in many aspects (the sexual and spiritual form) and provides for it an outlet so that those who seek true and unadulterated health can finally find fulfillment in all of the areas.

However, you do not have to have an imbalance of any sort to truly enjoy a tantric massage. While it is greatly beneficial to those who suffer, it is also beneficial to those who wish to ensure that their bodies stay aligned with the universe.

A tantric massage allows those who are shut off in their sexual lives to explore their sexual desires, enhance further sexual experiences, and become more comfortable with their sexuality in general.

In the tantric belief system, the prevailing idea is that humans were created to be uninhibited beings and that society, with its norms and its inherent guilt for things that are deemed "uncouth," have created inhibitions that we weren't naturally supposed to encounter and deal with. Tantric massages offer the option to get rid of those inhibitions and flush that guilt's out of our system so that we can become the being we were always meant to be.

As Tantra has evolved, it has drawn very steep correlations between sick and ill and the stipulations and stressors that society constantly bombards us with.

The idea is that, even though there were diseases that ran rampant for centuries before this, those studies have shown that those diseases were physically rooted in viruses and tangible reasons.

They teach that many of these psychological disabilities and chronic diseases have arisen with the add-ons and pressures of a morphing society. This alone has created a worldwide energy imbalance when attempting to connect to the life-force of the universe.

In other words: God (or gods) has created our bodies to experience intense sexual pleasure, and it makes no sense for that to be a part of our existence that is deprived because society has deemed it "inappropriate." Think about it: what if nourishing yourself with food was somehow deemed inappropriate. What if society began to teach that taking in as little food as possible would somehow make you a more acceptable person in society? There would be immense outrage and thousands of scientific studies pulled from the

shadows as to how this trend will wreak havoc on the human population.

And yet, it has been done to the needed sexual aspect of being human for decades.

Utilizing a tantric massage to awaken the seven energy centers that are cantered in various positions along the spine (which have been proven to exist because of the way our major nerve centers are set up along the body's spinal cord) can lead to overall sexual health, self-awareness, treatment for many chronic aches and pains, as well as provide coping mechanisms that can serve an individual well out in society.

 Focusing on the purely sexual aspect of a tantric massage and deeming it inappropriate is just as close-minded as taking a look at hunting and deeming it inappropriate for everyone because you feel that hunting one's meat is somehow inhumane.

A tantric massage has incredible benefits as well as freeing aspects that absolutely everyone can benefit from. If you can cast aside your skewed ideas of what you believe a tantric massage to be, a client can obtain an entirely different level of existing.

It can also give someone a different lens through which to view the world and a way to cope with past traumas that have prevented them from having fulfilling aspects of their own individual lives.

A tantric massage is a healing venture, not a sexual one. Just as society has bastardized several natural aspects of life, so it has bastardized the idea of a tantric massage.

The only true way you will ever be able to talk about it educationally is to study up on the beliefs and then experience one.

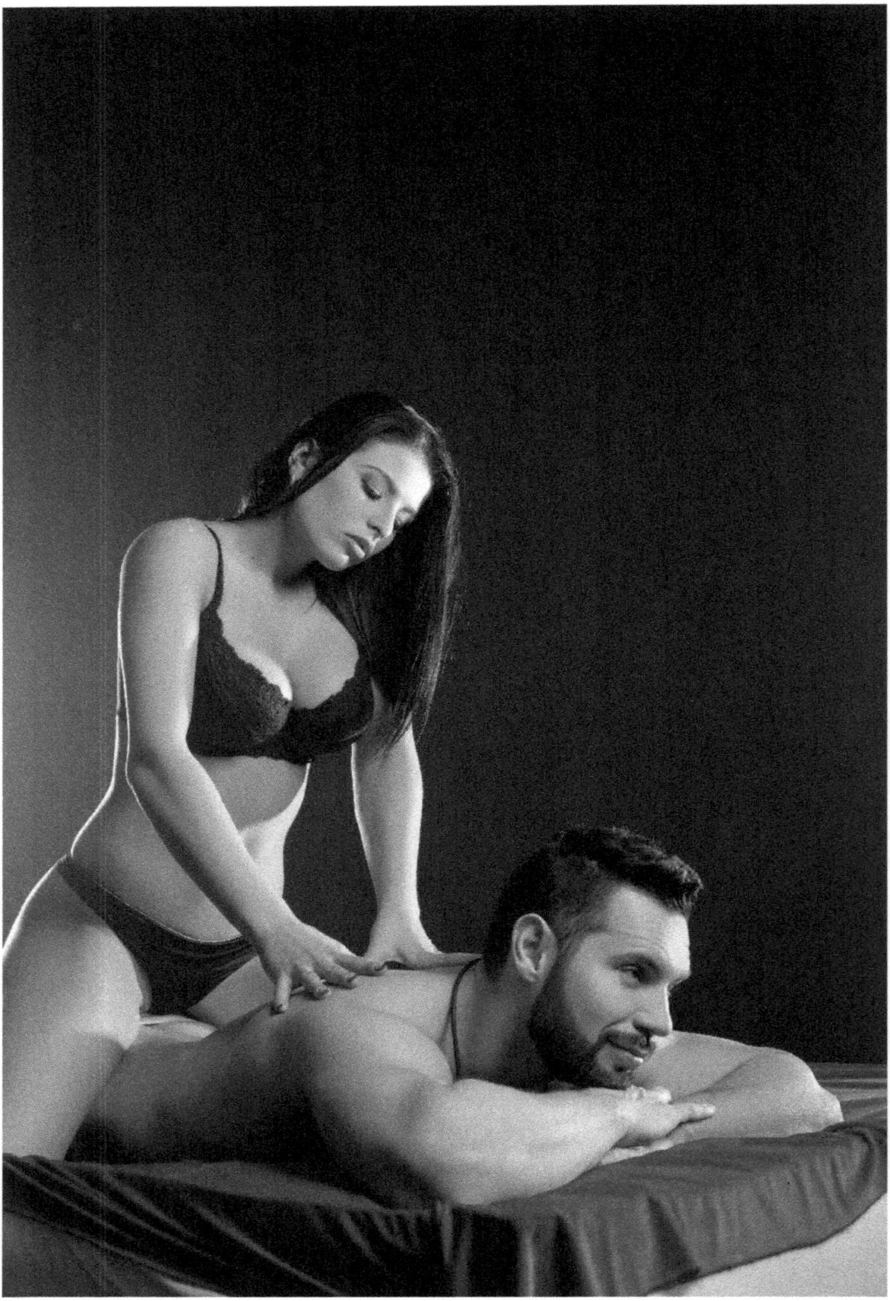

Conclusion

One of the primary principles of Tantra is there is no form of energy in the Universe that does not exist in our body.

Tantra also means technique, and it is that which helps us leverage the different forms of energy available in our body in a conscious way so that there is increased productivity in your life.

Although the secrets of the Tantra tradition were kept a secret for hundreds of years for multiple reasons, including the chances of them being misunderstood and misinterpreted, today, thanks to the internet and the world becoming a global village, more and more people are clearing their heads of misunderstandings and are given themselves to the magic of this system to lead a more fulfilled, happy, and healthy lifestyle than before.